The Hunger
Within

The Hunger Within

A Twelve-Week Guided Journey from Compulsive Eating to Recovery

Marilyn Ann Migliore

with Philip Ross

Main Street Books
Doubleday
New York   London   Toronto   Sydney   Auckland

A Main Street Book

PUBLISHED BY DOUBLEDAY
a division of Bantam Doubleday Dell Publishing Group, Inc.
1540 Broadway, New York, New York 10036

MAIN STREET BOOKS, DOUBLEDAY, and the portrayal of a building with a tree
are trademarks of Doubleday, a division of
Bantam Doubleday Dell Publishing Group, Inc.

Book design by Donna Sinisgalli

Library of Congress Cataloging-in-Publication Data

Migliore, Marilyn Ann.
The hunger within: a 12-week guided journey to recovery from
compulsive eating / Marilyn Ann Migliore, with Philip Ross.
p.   cm.
1. Compulsive eaters—Rehabilitation.   2. Compulsive eating—
Treatment.   3. Eating disorders—Treatment.   4. Food habits—
Psychological aspects.   5. Self-help techniques.   I. Ross. Philip.
II. Title.
RC552.C65M525   1998
616.85′26—dc21   98-41254
                                                                                            CIP

To the memory of

my brother, Greg,

whose spirit is with me

always

❧

Author's Note

❧

The material in this workbook has been constructed and presented in a way that will preserve the privacy and guarantee the confidentiality of my workshop participants. Thus, any resemblance to actual persons or events, living or dead, is entirely coincidental.

Contents

❧

PROLOGUE   ix

INTRODUCTION   xv

Stage One: Exploration

Week One: Welcome Aboard   3

Week Two: The Hunger Within   16

Week Three: Family Ties   34

Week Four: The Scariest Word   50

Stage Two: Discovery

Week Five: The Vicious Cycle   65

Week Six: Forbidden Fruit   81

Week Seven: Casting Call   96

Week Eight: Mirror, Mirror, on the Wall   112

Stage Three: Recovery

Week Nine: The Turning Point   133

Week Ten: Back to the Future   149

Week Eleven: Connections   170

Week Twelve: Beginning Again   183

SUGGESTED READING   197

Prologue

❧

Seated at a long oval table in a nondescript room on the ninth floor of an outpatient medical office building in Manhattan, a group of self-conscious adults are introducing themselves.

Fern describes herself in clipped tones as an attorney who is a partner in a small firm that specializes in real estate law. She is a graduate of Ivy League schools and has lived alone in the fifteen years since getting her first job. Unsurprisingly, the most intimate information Fern provides about herself concerns the reason she is here: "I have lost and gained more than five hundred pounds since my teens," she says, pain radiating from eyes that have receded into a fleshy face. "I have taken all kinds of diet pills and have been on six separate liquid diets. I have lost count of the number of weight-loss programs I've 'successfully' attended. I've come to think of dieting as my real profession. And although I realize that the vicious cycle of losing weight, then putting it back on plus some more, happens to more than ninety percent of dieters, that's hardly a consolation. I've never weighed as much as I weigh now, and I feel like I'm caught in a nightmarish maze with no exit."

Knowing nods from three or four women are punctured by a throaty male laugh. "Yeah, tell me about it," chortles Brendan, a mid-fortyish Falstaffian figure who, in every sense, seems larger than life. "If I only had a hundred bucks for every pound I've gained since I gave up drinking ten years ago, I could have invested it in this bull market and retired early." A stockbroker himself, Brendan leans back and tweaks his fireman's suspenders in obvious pleasure at the laughter he has elicited. One's first impressions are that he is a man of insatiable if not unquenchable appetites, who is gifted at lowering his own and others' anxieties through comic self-mockery. Indeed, in the next couple of minutes, Brendan reels off his unsuccessful battles in the pasta wars, his medical woes, his doctor's warnings, in so entertaining a fashion that we are all reduced to giggles and guffaws by someone who is telling us he could keel over any day now.

Brendan would be a hard act to follow for anyone, but perhaps more so for Mary, the homemaker turned nurse after the last of her four children left for college. Hidden inside a drab dress purchased joylessly from a catalogue that specializes in euphemistic names for obesity, Mary looks as if she'd give anything for a place to hide. When she speaks, it is in the hushed voice of a penitent making confession. She lists the years of eating "sins" that have turned her into the "fatty," as she puts it, that we see today. She mentions that most of her overeating has occurred at night, after taking care of her kids and husband, and more recently, of the patients on her hospital shift. She says that food has been her reward, but that her "just desserts" are causing her, among other things, sore joints. Wistfully, she notes that she is no longer able to join her husband in hiking and other outdoor activities they used to enjoy together.

Others share their own short stories, all of which revolve around food and their problematic relationship with it. For all their differences, these people share much more in common than excess pounds. They are all bright. They don't need to be told that a cup of broccoli has fewer calories than a cup of Häagen-Dazs.

They may talk about the temptations of leftovers, about jobs that require lots of dining out, of sweet tooths or problems around the holidays, but on some level they also know it's about none of these things. Fern will understandably make no reference today to her mother's expectations, Brendan to his father's beatings, or Mary to the woman's name and phone number she found last week scribbled on a piece of paper in her husband's trousers. They will talk only about food. Some will actually identify themselves as compulsive eaters.

Perhaps most important, the people sitting around this table today, like the hundreds who have come before them, are fellow travelers on the dieting roller coaster, people whose losing battles have filled them not only with excess pounds but with shame, inadequacy, and self-loathing. They, like you, may not be able to articulate it, but religious or not, they are here in a desperate attempt to save their souls.

If you've picked up this book and have read this far, chances are you know all too well that for most people, including yourself, diets don't work! You have tried different programs. You have read through what seem like a zillion books and magazines about weight, and have ended up at best confused and discouraged, at worst resigned. One magazine tells you to count fat grams and avoid carbohydrates. Another tells you to eat all the chocolate you want. A miracle drug promises to help you drop ten pounds in a week. The latest gastronomical guru says the whole secret is combining Food A with Food B.

And none of it works! None of it works because, for compulsive eaters, nutritional information, good, bad, or indifferent, is irrelevant. You already know that if you take in more calories than you expend, you will gain weight, and vice versa. You know how to count calories when you want to count calories. Not only do you know that exercise is good for you, but you could probably determine without too much difficulty how walking a mile at a twenty-minute pace compares calorically with fifteen minutes on a Stairmaster at Level 3.

All this information is, I repeat, irrelevant. For compulsive eaters, the problem is not lack of information about food or exercise. Food is not the issue. The issue, as you are all too well aware, is the repetitive nature of your compulsive behavior, or what I call your *life script,* when it comes to the interplay of food and feelings.

What you don't understand is why or how. *Why* you are stuck in compulsive behaviors that make you unable to eat the way you imagine "normal" people do. *How* to get out of this emotional quagmire.

In a world filled with psychobabble, it's easy for the meaning of words to be lost. So let me be clear from the outset about what I mean when I refer to compulsive eating. When I use that term, I am talking about any kind of non-hunger-related eating acted out in a repetitive fashion that leads to negative physical and emotional consequences.

Compulsive eating has been compared with sharks on a feeding frenzy. Just listen to the words I've heard my workshop participants use to describe their binges:

"I shoveled the gallon of ice cream into my mouth so quickly that

I barely gave myself a chance to breathe. When it was over, I retreated into my bedroom, overwhelmed with feelings of shame."

"I stared at the television set, transfixed like a zombie. It was like I was in a trance. I was completely unaware of what my hands were doing or of the mounting pile of candy wrappers at my feet."

"From the time I entered the supermarket—actually from some point earlier than that—it was as though I had entered, or was pulled, into this strange zone. It felt almost like a gravitational force was drawing me into its orbit and that I was heading for oblivion."

Recognize yourself?

When a compulsive eater enters the "trance state" that precedes and accompanies an eating binge, an encyclopedia of nutritional information will turn to instant mush. Telling a compulsive eater that finishing off the key lime pie in the refrigerator will result in so many calories is like telling someone in the middle of a sex act that without percautions, pregnancy or disease might result. Chances are the person has not gotten to this point because of an educational deficiency. How many of you reading this, for example, are thinking, "If only someone had told me that the five slices of pizza with sausages I devoured last night had more calories than what I used up during the half hour it took me to eat them while watching that rerun of Mary Tyler Moore?"

It's knowing the answers and not acting on them that makes you feel so desperate!

It doesn't have to be that way.

If the tone of this book is confident, it is because I have witnessed success with people who have struggled most of their lives with food, eating, and weight issues. When they come to my workshop, they finally feel they have found something that is taking them in the right direction. I am also confident because the journey you are about to embark upon is guided by some of the most contemporary research and thinking in the treatment of compulsive eating. But before we set out, a friendly word of warning: If your focus is simply on quick weight loss, this is not the book for you. There are, as I've said, tons of programs and printed material giving you new diets every year.

On the other hand, although this book will not spell out a diet plan for you or treat the symptom that is your excess weight, your body invariably will begin to normalize as you begin to make the emotional changes that lie at the heart of *The Hunger Within*.

Most important, this is not simply a book. It's an interactive *work-book* designed exclusively for compulsive eaters. It is filled with exercises and information that will help you explore and subdue the forces driving your eating patterns. This workbook will serve as a road map, an encouraging companion you can turn to again and again. By following the steps laid out in the pages ahead, you will learn what your life script is all about. You will come to understand how the initial messages you received in your formative years and the way you interpreted them came to shape the major themes of your life drama.

Together, we can rewrite the script so that compulsive eating recedes from center stage to an occasional cameo appearance at most.

Ready? I hope so, because we're about to set out together on an exhilarating journey. It is a journey you will not be traveling alone. Fern, Brendan, Mary, and I will be walking each step with you. We will share each other's laughter, tears, excitement, and revelations as we meet each task head on, in search of *The Hunger Within*.

Introduction

❧

If you were to go on a photo safari in Africa, you would probably experience firsthand the drama of the hunter and the prey. You might see a pride of lionesses giving chase to a zebra or a pack of hyenas hard on the heels of a young warthog. As you watched this primal scene, you would understand implicitly that a story was being written based on a genetic script. The lions, for example, are doing what lions do. The possibility that one day a lioness may pause, contemplate her navel, and suggest to her fellow felines that "maybe this carnivore thing isn't all it's cracked up to be" is about as likely as the zebra announcing that he has a sudden craving for a water-buffalo burger.

When it comes to food choices, other species operate out of a genetic mandate, which, I might note, does not include compulsive eating. With us, it's different. We are the only living creatures who can step out of the river of life, look at ourselves, come to conclusions, and make choices. Choices which, in turn, create change. And although "change" may be the scariest word in the English language, it is something we yearn for when we are stuck in a cycle of self-destructive behavior.

I understand that for the compulsive eater, the trance state during a binge may be so powerful that it may seem as inevitable as the lioness tearing into a fresh kill. I'm here to tell you it's not.

When we eat compulsively, we are not playing out a genetic role, but enacting what I call an emotional script. The script is unconscious.

It was invariably written during our early, developmental years. Other players were involved. And the collaboration determined the relationship we would have with food in the years to come.

Of course, you already know this! You know that when you eat compulsively, there is some intense relationship going on between food and feelings. You probably don't know a whole lot about this intimate experience, but you are familiar with it in every sense of the word.

You also believe, I'm sure, that the unconscious plays an important part in our daily lives, and not just in negative ways. You might, for example, find yourself reading a book and listening to some music and suddenly something comes on that has you on your feet and dancing. Perhaps at the moment you're not sure why this particular song has had this effect, but you know it's about more than music. And perhaps only later will you remember that evening oh so many years ago, when you were sitting in a café during a romantic evening and this was the song that was being played. So this experience you're having seems to be about music, but is really about something very different.

And so it is when it comes to our relationship with food. When compulsive eaters talk about their *loss of connection* to themselves and their environment during a feeding frenzy, it is because they have been *reconnected* to a whole set of unconscious links between feelings and food. The problem is, while the music may open up feelings that take you back to some lovely time and place, the unconscious feelings/food relationship that is regularly triggered leads you down the path of despair.

The Hunger Within is going to help you change the script. During the twelve weeks or more we're going to spend together, we'll write a new one that will enable you to take control of your eating. Along with Fern, Brendan, and Mary, you will find out how the old script was generated. Using a series of simple, experiential daily exercises, you will bring the unconscious to the surface. If you are willing to put in a little effort, you can discover the key to permanently unlocking the self-imprisoning features of your life script.

The exercises in this book are easy to follow, and many who have participated in my program say they are actually enjoyable in the unique way self-discovery can be liberating. You may even want to form your own group so that the feedback and reinforcement you get from me and the workshop participants I describe can be enhanced by a live, shared experience.

The program has three stages. Each has four parts.

Week One marks the beginning of the Exploration Stage. You will start to get up close and personal with compulsive eating, not as an abstract concept or a national statistic, but through Fern, Brendan, and Mary. Through them, you will begin to discover how food, dieting, and eating come into play in one's life script. A questionnaire and exercises will help you make some connections for yourself.

Then in Week Two, along with Fern, Brendan, and Mary, you will begin to explore the origins of compulsive eating. You will learn how *psychological* hunger forms the foundation on which disordered eating builds. Exercises will help you identify the *emotional climate* that dictates the direction of your script.

In Week Three, our growing awareness of the psychological hunger we experienced early in our lives allows us now to begin to identify the *early decisions* we made about ourselves and the world around us. We will see how these decisions set the major themes for our script. To see how food and feelings figure into this, we will create family maps, or *genograms,* to get to the roots of our eating behaviors.

As I've said, the scariest word is "change," and in Week Four you will learn why. As you get ready to bid farewell to Stage One, it is of vital importance that you understand why you hold on to your script so tenaciously. Side by side with Fern, Brendan, and Mary, you will pay homage to your *resistance* to pressing the "delete" button on your emotional computer. A few safe experiments will prove to you what I mean.

By Week Five we are in the Discovery Stage. This is the time to bring out the looking glass and see beyond it to events in your life and to the meaning you attach to them. You will begin to identify the feelings that invariably flow from those thoughts, how feeling turns to feeding, and, amazingly, how the compulsive eating completes the loop and reaffirms your self-image.

Week Six: Hold on to your emotional hats! We're going to be eating potato chips. We're going to be eating chocolate. We're going to be sticking the "bad" food right in our mouths, and we're going to see just where *demystifying* food takes us. And by Week Seven you will be invited to a private performance of a drama that has been playing in your mind for a very long time. You will meet the all-star cast, also known as your family. You will discover how well you know *their* roles. You will see how many of their lines you have memorized. In Week Eight you'll get them interacting, all those characters you know so well. As you hold them up to the mirror, you will have much to reflect on as you experience directly how they communicate.

Week Nine marks the beginning of the Recovery Stage. During this week, you will begin to make peace with the cast of characters that have been playing in your head and perpetuating the compulsive features of your life script.

Your efforts will be rewarded in Week Ten. You have taken a long, hard, and honest look at your triggers and patterns. You will be ready to begin making your way out of the jungle. The only map you'll need is a photograph of yourself as a child. You'll be introduced to a new guide here, and she will take you by the hand and walk you in the right direction.

Week Eleven is where you bring to bear everything you've learned as you create a powerful intervention to help yourself on the last leg of your journey to recovery.

Finally, in Week Twelve, we'll do a quick review to make sure you're where you want to be. We'll look to the future to anticipate possible danger zones and plan interventions. And, finally, we'll say goodbye. At least for now.

While *The Hunger Within* is laid out as a twelve-week itinerary, the time frame is not important. Progress at your own pace. You may want to stay in one chapter for a week or several weeks before moving on.

What is important is that you take yourself seriously enough to make sure you have some time each day, preferably the same time, when there are no distractions and you have privacy. Most weeks include one or more exercises for you to participate in as you read along. At the end of every week, you'll also find a heading called Food for Thought. This essential component of the workbook consists of daily writing tasks for you to complete and the space to do them. These "homework" assignments can be the key to your success. They will help you reflect on the reading. They will give you a chance to practice what you've learned. They will keep you focused.

Don't be discouraged if you find yourself at an impasse, say, at Week Four. Chapters progress developmentally, and it may help your development to go back to weeks one, two, or three and reuse the material there to gain the confidence you need to move ahead.

Finally, be aware that because you will actively, or *experientially,* participate in each chapter, you will be tapping in to a part of yourself you may not have consciously accessed before. This is one other reason there surely will be times you need to pause and catch your breath before writing new chapters into your own life.

Stage One

❧

Exploration

Welcome Aboard

❧

In this first week, you will find that you do not dine alone at the table of compulsive eating. You will begin to understand how food fits in to the menu of your life.

I'd like to begin by introducing you to someone I hope you get to know much better in the weeks to come: *you.*

What follows are a bunch of statements that relate to you and food. Without taking too much time to think about each one, place a check in the space provided at the beginning of each statement that seems to apply.

_√_ 1. I frequently find myself preoccupied with thoughts of eating and food.

_√_ 2. I am typically self-conscious when eating in public.

___ 3. All things considered, I would prefer to eat alone.

_√_ 4. I eat secretly.

_√_ 5. I tend to consume huge amounts of food in short periods of time.

___ 6. I find that afterward I don't remember exactly how I ate all that food.

_√_ 7. If tempting foods are in my home, I won't rest until I've eaten them.

8. My past efforts to control my eating have failed.
9. Before I head for the refrigerator, I am sometimes aware of feelings like loneliness or anxiety.
10. Before and during my rendezvous with food, I experience a temporary sense of comfort.
11. I usually feel guilty after I've consumed the food.
12. My sense of self-worth is intimately connected to my weight.

Restlessness and discontent are the necessities of progress.

—THOMAS EDISON

There is no need to turn the above into a pseudoscientific exercise by asking you to tally up your responses and coming up with a formula, e.g., "If you put checks after six or more statements . . ." The plain truth is—and I don't think you need much convincing on this point—that if you're a compulsive eater, you found yourself in almost all of these statements. And if you are as reluctant to label yourself a compulsive eater as a drinker is to call himself an alcoholic, welcome to the crowd. Who among us, after all, likes the idea of acknowledging to ourselves, much less to anyone else, that we're out of control?

Perhaps Mary, the housewife turned nurse whom you met in the Prologue, put it best when compulsive eating came up in the first week of my workshop: "This is a subject," she said with quiet intensity, "that I really wish I didn't have to talk about."

On second thought, perhaps we *should* linger for a few moments before labeling ourselves compulsive eaters. If the drinker finds solace in the idea that he has a bit too much from time to time, but nothing more, then it's certainly understandable that the eater would take comfort in the idea that she overindulges in food, perhaps regularly, but not compulsively. The distinction between *overeating* and *compulsive eating,* I assure you, is not merely academic. If you're an occasional overeater, a few little tips are probably all you need and you're on your way. You know, drink more water; step up the exercise; keep away from late-night eating. Compulsive eating, on the other hand, is a cake of a different batter. It may look like regular chocolate cake on the outside, but the ingredients are not at all the same. Let's use drinking to help flesh out the difference. Take two men. One comes home every evening and has a drink before dinner. The other comes home every night and can't have dinner without first having a drink. Each man drinks the same amount, yet the second is dependent on alcohol. There is a compulsive quality to his drinking. He is, in fact, an alcoholic.

Who cares about the difference if each guy is having one drink? Good point! The problem is, in real life the alcoholic doesn't have just one drink any more than the compulsive eater has just one cookie. Remember Brendan, the stockbroker with the gift of gab you met earlier? Here's the way he put it: "When I drank, a fly climbing up a wall could be reason enough to break out the bottle. It's the same now with food. Every night is a special occasion. First I have my dinner. Sometime later, I sit down to eat."

The eating Brendan is talking about arises out of a powerful impulse that seems too much to resist. It has the same all-consuming pull as the physical addiction of heroin or nicotine. Like these drugs, the food fix offers the same temporary solace, or relief, followed by a cycle of shame and guilt. And just as inevitably, before long the urge to binge returns again and cannot be denied. The vicious cycle of *obsessive thoughts* leading to *compulsive behavior* has all the predictability of any long-established ritual. Unlike many other rituals, however, we experience these eating episodes on a largely unconscious level. We go into "automatic" in much the same way as we might stop at a red light or step on the gas when it turns green.

A great example of how this ritualistic, compulsive eating works was described by Fern, the attorney whom you also met in the Prologue. When Fern heard me use the expression "going on automatic," she was courageous enough to offer up the following story from her own life:

"Last week, I went into an automobile dealer to buy a new car. I had really done my homework. I had studied *Consumer Reports* and chosen the make, the model, and the options I wanted. I had read about different negotiating strategies. I had done everything right, but when the salesman and I got down to hard-nosed bargaining and he began to laugh when I talked and started calling me 'honey,' I really lost it. I felt humiliated. He damn well wouldn't have done that with a man. Sometime on the way home, I began thinking about the supermarket. I remember consciously thinking that I needed some milk and cat food and a couple of other things, but at some point while I was walking down the aisles, I began thinking about the frozen-food section. I don't think I was really conscious of why, or what was going on when I arrived, but I know that when I was checking out a few minutes later, one of the things being loaded into my shopping bag was a quart of ice cream.

Venus yields to caresses, not to compulsion.

—PUBLILIUS SYRUS

"But that's only the beginning of the automatic part of what happened. The next is that when I got home, it was early enough for me to watch Oprah, and—this is so ironic I can hardly believe it—the show was on losing weight, and I sat there taking in all the opinions, and when it was over I looked down and saw maybe three or four teaspoons' worth of ice cream left in that quart container. And let me tell you, if I felt bad about what happened at the automobile dealer, this didn't exactly make me feel better about myself."

Brendan related to Fern's experience: "I've been in plenty of humiliating situations in my life. The worst were when I was a kid. And I know how terrible it is to feel you haven't stood up for yourself or that you can't. I also know all about what happened with Fern and food afterward. I used to use alcohol to blot out feelings, and I'm sure that's what I do now with food. But as I said before, I don't really need some negative event to set me off. I can binge regularly, and I can do it after I've had a perfectly fine day."

"That confuses me too," Fern added. "I gave that example, but I have big issues around food no matter what. I know I rarely eat because I'm hungry. When I'm having dinner with a girlfriend and I see her put her fork down with food still left on her plate and say, 'That was delicious, but I'm stuffed,' she might as well be a Martian. That's how alien she seems to me."

For Mary, Fern's story rang a different bell. "It's the secrecy of the whole thing," Mary said. "Not just the part of eating a quart of ice cream alone, which I would never do in front of someone else, but also the way Fern seems to have kept the buying and eating of the ice cream a secret from herself. Of course, I also know exactly how Fern felt about herself after she had finished the ice cream. It doesn't exactly make you proud of yourself."

If you're a compulsive eater, you've not only found ways to relate to Fern's story, but you know what all three are talking about when they express the urgency to eat as a highly charged emotional issue.

To give yourself a taste of just how emotional an issue food is for you and how disconnected it is from hunger, I'd like to suggest the following exercise: Pick a time when you have the urge to eat. Dinner would be a good time. Now, all I'd like you to do is *not* finish everything on your plate. I mean, just leave a *little* there. Maybe a couple of forkfuls of pasta, or the right-hand corner of that piece of bread. Better yet, leave a quarter of your dessert untouched. That's right, just

You cannot create experience. You must undergo it.

—ALBERT CAMUS

sitting there while the others finish theirs. If that seems too much, eat everything and don't take seconds when the serving dishes are being passed around.

I want you to pay careful attention to yourself while you are abstaining, to become intimately familiar with your impulse to eat. Remember, you should be reasonably full when you leave a little pasta or pie on your plate or when you say no to seconds. For someone with no major emotional issues around food, saying no to seconds should be as casual a decision as saying no to another glass of wine would be to a casual drinker or turning down an opportunity to bet on the Kentucky Derby would be to a nongambler.

Think about the kinds of feelings you had during dinner. Was saying no a casual experience? It sure wasn't for Fern, Brendan, and Mary. "It just proved my point about people not finishing what's on their plate being like Martians to me," Fern reported heatedly the next week. "Only this time I joined the Martians and it was terrible. I was out for dinner with my brother, and I decided I wouldn't eat part of my dinner roll, and as we moved from salad to the main course to coffee, I kept glancing down at that little piece of roll I hadn't touched and it was agony. I was so distracted that I couldn't even concentrate on what my brother was saying half the time. It seems so crazy. What on earth could that little piece of roll have offered me that I should be so focused on it?"

Brendan put it in his own inimitable way. "Marilyn, I wanted to kill you," he said laughing. "I was at a business dinner with a client whom I've made a lot of money for in the market and who has made a lot of money for me in commissions. We're sitting there having a great time, telling jokes, and I don't know why, but it occurs to me to do the homework now, so I decide I won't finish my blueberry pie, and I'm sitting there and sitting there, and after a while, I swear I've decided that you're a sadist—that you have created this assignment for the sole purpose of torturing me. Casual? You've got to be kidding!"

Mary expressed her discomfort less exuberantly. "I decided not to have any more of the roast potatoes I had made for dinner after my husband had taken seconds himself and passed the bowl to me. What did it feel like? Nothing, really. I wasn't in any kind of pain or anything, but if I'm honest with myself, I have to admit that I knew my husband would be in the den watching sports later and I was already thinking about my late-night snack."

Adversity is the first path to truth.

—Lord Byron

What Fern, Brendan, and Mary are talking about, of course, is not food but their *obsession* with food. The obsession part of what you go through is what you experience *before* you begin to eat or *while* you're consciously refraining. It's the combination of recurring, unwanted thoughts and images and feelings of distress. I should hasten to add that almost all of us experience obsessive thoughts on occasion. That's normal (and by "normal" I am talking about statistics, not making moral or value judgments). What's not normal is having obsessive thoughts about food all the time. Compulsive eaters seem unable to stop the obsessing. The more they try, the more the unwanted thoughts keep flooding back. And when your thoughts are so all-consuming, it's virtually impossible to be present, to be *here*. You tend to feel disconnected from other people *and* from yourself. No wonder you feel so alone.

That's where the *compulsion* part kicks in. It's the repetitive ritual that the person has unconsciously invented (with great creativity when you come to think about it) to make the obsessions go away, to destroy those uncomfortable, circular thoughts, and, most important, to keep you away from the true hunger that lies within.

If you're obsessed about food and eating, it makes sense that eating a whole lot of food will take care of the obsessive thoughts. Eighty percent of people with obsessive thoughts, as a matter of fact, say that by performing specific rituals or behaviors, they *do* feel better—temporarily. And that's the problem. For the compulsive eater, the obsession with food followed by the feeding frenzy *does* provide temporary relief, but the relief doesn't last much longer than the time it takes to consume the food. Then the cycle begins all over again.

That the solution is only temporary is not the only problem, of course. There are also the practical consequences that result from a particular solution. For the drinker there are dozens of consequences, ranging from cirrhosis of the liver to becoming violent to running over a child while driving drunk. The compulsive gambler may lose his home and job. The sex "addict" may contract deadly diseases. The drug user may end up in jail. For the compulsive eater the practical consequences go beyond appearances and self-image. The health implications of the excess pounds your compulsive eating creates, from your ankles to your aorta, are profound.

"I'm a nurse, and I know all about obesity and health," Mary says, "but as we've each agreed, information doesn't seem to help. After all, people who smoke know it's bad for them, but that doesn't mean they're going to stop."

"We also know diets don't work," Fern chips in, "but that doesn't stop millions of people from going on new ones every year."

"That's because people want a quick cure," says Brendan. "The same thing happens in the investing business when people lose their savings because they get taken in by some hot stock that they think is going to make them rich overnight."

"I think the reason diets don't work is because they treat the symptom, or the weight, and not the cause," Mary says. "It's like treating internal bleeding by giving the patient a massage. For me, a good example of this is that in the first years after my marriage, I didn't eat compulsively. I cleaned compulsively. We had bought a new house, and—there is no other word for it—I was *obsessed* with cleaning it and keeping everything neat. I would go into a frenzy if things were out of place. I was so preoccupied that friends began to notice, and although they were always complimenting me, a few expressed concerns. They worried that I was going above and beyond, and that I seemed to be running myself ragged in the process. And it's only today, sitting here, that I realize that when I started to eat compulsively, my cleaning became less obsessive."

What's going on here?

"I don't have a clue," Brendan says, "but I think I must be related to Mary, because my weight started to increase after I quit drinking. Before, I felt bad about how much Chivas Regal I drank. Now it's how much cheesecake I ate."

"I can top both Brendan and Mary," Fern commiserates. "There was a time in my life, maybe twelve or so years ago, when I was on a diet and I actually reached my goal weight. And guess what? Soon after, I was spending an hour a day or more checking to make sure that my door was locked and my phone wasn't off the hook. Finally I sought help and was diagnosed as having an obsessive-compulsive disorder. This was before they treated this with medication, and the talk therapy wasn't working. And do you know what the cure was? Food! As soon as I began to eat compulsively again and gain weight, I stopped being anxious about the door or the phone."

What's going on here is that in substituting compulsions Mary and Brendan and Fern are changing deck chairs on the *Titanic*. And, as in a good mystery, things are not what they seem to be. The most obvious suspect turns out not to be the real villain. In the mystery of com-

Every soul is a melody which needs renewing.

—STÉPHANE MALLARMÉ

pulsive eating, the prime suspect is food, and food, we shall see, is just a red herring.

What function does food serve for you?

Fern: "I don't have a clue. All I know is that when I come home from work, I have to have something—food or a drink—in my hands at all times or I'll start climbing the walls."

Brendan: "You talked about compulsive behavior providing temporary relief, and there's no question about it, I feel calmer when I'm eating."

Mary: "I keep thinking about the part that involves secrecy. I don't know why, but I have this strong feeling that for me, secrecy plays a big role."

Those who dare to fail miserably can achieve greatly.

—ROBERT KENNEDY

This is not a question I expect you to explore fully now. I want to introduce it at this time only because I've been taking pains to point out that compulsive eating isn't about food any more than compulsive cleaning is about dirty floors. The key word in the question, "What function does food serve for you?" is "function." When something has a function, it has a *purpose* or *use.*

In Arthur Miller's classic play *Death of a Salesman,* the tragically flawed protagonist, Willy Loman, is defended at one point by his wife. Yes, she says, Willy has obvious faults, but his virtues should not be overlooked. "Attention must be paid!" she demands.

Let us now pay attention to the virtues of compulsive eating. Yes, *virtues.* What I'd like you to do below is make a list of all the positive functions you can imagine that food and your preoccupation with it serve. The quotes above from Mary, Brendan, and Fern were the first thoughts that came into their minds. How about you? List anything you can think of that in its own way might work for you to go into a food trance and disconnect from yourself and the world around you.

_____

_____

_____

_____

Over the next week, when you reach for food, I'd like you to ask yourself, "What function is this food serving for me at this moment?" Keep notes if you can.

When I asked Mary what function compulsive eating served for her, you may recall, she said she thought the secrecy of the act had something to do with it. Exactly what, we'll be investigating with a fine-tooth comb in later weeks. For now, I'd like to underline Mary's intuition. Secrecy usually goes with compulsive eating like, well, peanut butter goes with jelly. We can't carry on our illicit affair with food if others are watching—or if we're aware that they're watching. Sometimes we can't even do it if *we're* watching! That's why we go into a trance state and disconnect, whether we're alone or in the grand ballroom of a wedding party.

What would your life be like if food were not a focus?

If your obsession with food serves some kind of function, then the question on the table is, What would your life be like if food were not a focus? It's a question I'd like you to ask yourself now. How would things be different? When I posed this question to my workshop participants, here's what they said:

Brendan: "I'd be more physically active—and that includes indoor sports!"

Mary: "I wish I could think of something positive. The only word that comes to mind is 'panicked.' I wish I could imagine something besides a great void."

Fern: "It's strange. I have no idea why, but the first thing that came into my mind is that I would be easier and kinder."

Now it's your turn. In the space below describe what you think *your* life would be like if food were not a focus.

_____

_____

_____

_____

You must do the thing you think you cannot do.

—Eleanor Roosevelt

HERE'S LOOKING AT YOU

To experience what it feels like to be *connected* with food, I have some homework for you. Sometime during the next week, I want you to eat while looking in a mirror. My sense is that you will balk at the idea, but bear with me. I promise that you will be okay and that it will enable you to get a new perspective. Watch yourself eat. Your face. Your mouth. Your utensils picking up the food. Keep watching. Take no notes. Just eat. And watch.

You are probably still dubious. You are not alone. Here were some first reactions from the participants in my workshop:

Fern: "No way! When I go into a restaurant, I never, ever, allow myself to be seated facing a mirror."

Brendan: "That's the way it was when I drank. I would always take the seat at the end of the bar where the mirror couldn't reach me."

Mary: "I'm going to be honest with you. I'm not sure I can do this."

This brings us to the end of our first week together, but for you it should be only the end of the beginning. What follows are a series of one-day writing and other exercises to take you through the week. They are your mental gym, and, like physical workouts, if you stick with them you'll see results.

It is only in adventure that some people succeed in knowing themselves . . . in finding themselves.

—ANDRÉ GIDE

FOOD FOR THOUGHT

WEEK ONE

Day One

How old were you when you went on your first diet? _____

Whose idea was it? _____

If it wasn't yours, how did you react? _____

What kind of a diet was it? _____

How long were you on it? _____

What were the results? _____

Create a graph that represents your past weight loss attempts.
What patterns do you see?

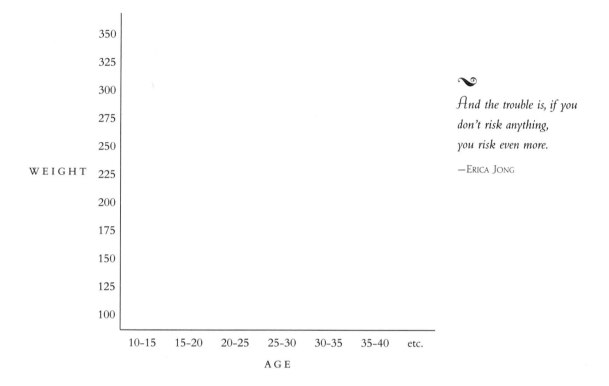

Day Two

In what ways are you secretive with food?
Buying: _____

_____

Storing: _____

_____

Eating: _____

Who are you hiding from? _____

What happens when you get caught? _____

_____

What do you say? _____
_____

What do you feel? _____
_____

Day Three

In what ways do you find yourself preoccupied with food?
Type of food: _____
Time of day: _____
Your thoughts: _____

Day Four

Describe your eating rituals. Try to be very specific.
Where do you usually eat? _____
Are you sitting or standing? _____
Do you use utensils? _____
Are you alone? _____
If a film were made of one of your eating binges, describe as visually as
possible what the audience would see. _____
_____

Day Five

Do you find yourself being self-conscious around food in public?
Describe how you show it.
When you are buying food: _____
When you are ordering food: _____
When you are eating out: _____

Day Six

What excuses do you find yourself making regarding:
The foods you purchase: _____
The foods you order in: _____
The foods you select from a restaurant menu: _____
The foods you bring into the house: _____

*Come,
and trip it,
as you go,
On the light fantastic toe.*

—JOHN MILTON

Day Seven

In what ways do you find yourself being compulsive other than with food?_____

_____

Describe:_____

_____

Weekly Checklist

___ 1. Did you complete the mirror exercise this week?
___ 2. Were you able to leave some food on your plate at mealtimes?
___ 3. Did you complete the Food for Thought exercises?

You may be disappointed if you fail, you are doomed if you don't try.

—BEVERLY SILLS

The Hunger Within

❧

This week you will learn about the three different kinds of hunger, how to tell them apart, and which one leads you to the refrigerator door.

❧

It seems to me that our three basic needs, for food and security and love, are so mixed and mingled and entwined that we cannot straightly think of one without the others.

—M. F. K. FISHER

Before moving on, let's go back for a few moments to last week. There were several experiences you tried on for size. You experimented with not eating everything on your plate. You wrote down the advantages of being obsessed with food. You thought about what freedom from that obsession might mean in your life. And finally, you ate a meal while looking at yourself in the mirror. What I hope you take away from all this is a heightened sense of how emotional an issue food is for you.

Fern, Brendan, and Mary sure did.

Fern: "I took a small portion so I could get through it quickly. I could barely stand to look at myself. It made me so self-conscious. And, of course, it was only a few minutes later, away from the mirror, that I began to eat in my 'regular' way."

Brendan: "Ditto for me. I couldn't wait to be done. There's something about being forced to look at yourself, to what you called staying connected, that changes everything."

Mary: "I agree, but I'm not sure in my case how much I hated it was because I wasn't eating 'on automatic' or because of how much I don't like the puffed-up face in the mirror."

❧

I hope that you'll go back from time to time to your responses in Week One. It will help you in many ways to stay in touch with who you are when it comes to eating, to keep reminding yourself that most of what you put in your mouth is about feelings, not food.

We began by talking about how lions are following a genetic script when they hunt and eat meat instead of grazing on grasslands. There's another thing about lions and almost all other kinds of animals: If left on their own, *they will eat when they're hungry.*

It's an amazing thing to watch animals in the wild eat. A pride of lionesses stalks a prey, makes a kill, then literally tears into the feast. When they are done, they sleep, play, mate. Sometimes you will see them walking in a casual file not far from a herd of zebras or other potential prey. The lionesses make no move to attack. The zebras continue munching. They show virtually no fear. Why? Because the lionesses are not hungry and the zebras *know it.* On another occasion, the zebras would be running for their lives. This time they can relax and let the feared felines walk on by.

What we have just witnessed in nature is a collaboration in which two species of animals know when one of them is hungry. How does a lioness know when she's hungry? What cues does the zebra pick up? Interesting questions to ask if you're heading for the Serengeti, but not nearly as fascinating as the question I'm going to ask you now:

How do you know when you're hungry?

Fern: "I almost never eat when I'm truly hungry in a physical sense. Maybe on occasion when I've been tied up with some work in the office and I can hear my stomach growl. Oh, yes, I'm Jewish, and on the holiday of Yom Kippur, I fast for twenty-four hours. Then I get a real sense of what it means to be hungry."

Brendan: "You don't have to be Jewish to like eating when you're not physically hungry. I can't remember the last time I heard my stomach growl. I'd settle for a little meow. I'm not really hungry when I have my muffin in the morning because I've eaten so much the night before. We always go out for lunch before I'm really hungry. I usually have an afternoon doughnut or something off the snack cart that makes the rounds. And by early evening, I'm into my Hall of Fame eating."

❧

And he said: you pretty full of yourself ain't chu. So she replied: show me someone not full of herself and I'll show you a hungry person.

—NIKKI GIOVANNI

Mary: "Being a nurse, I know that true hunger is related to a drop in blood sugar. I remember learning that when your blood sugar drops, the cells in your central nervous system detect this and react. Like the others here, I have very little personal experience of what it's like, but I recall a couple of years ago when I had to fast before a blood test, I began to feel dizzy."

P H Y S I C A L   H U N G E R

A journey of a thousand miles must begin with a single step.

—CHINESE PROVERB

The first of the three forms of hunger, what some call "true" or "real" hunger, is physical hunger. In the absence of food for a sufficient period of time, we develop physical symptoms. Mary is right when she mentions dizziness as one of these symptoms. But how about that stomach growling Fern and Brendan talked about? Isn't stomach growling the surest sign? To take a line from *Porgy and Bess,* it ain't necessarily so.

Studies show that the stomach actually has its own "brain," and secretes the same neurotransmitters as the brain in our head. Moreover, the stomach also experiences *feelings.* The heart is the organ we usually associate with feelings. When it comes to organic metaphors, the stomach gets short shrift. Since we give the heart the high road, the maligned stomach is left with "I can't stomach that" and "I had butterflies in my stomach" and "That was a gut-wrenching experience" and "My stomach was tied up in knots."

Truth is, we ought to be sending out cards shaped like stomachs, because the stomach, unlike the heart, does experience feelings. When your stomach is growling, you are secreting gastric juices. If you put your hand on your stomach when that happens, you can actually feel the rumbling sensation. Now, this *might* mean that we're physically hungry, but the acid we're secreting might also mean we're anxious, or experiencing some other form of stress. So the stomach, unfortunately, is not always an accurate barometer for letting us know whether our blood sugar is dropping and we're running short of body fuel. Other signs of physical hunger include lightheadedness, headache, fatigue, decreased concentration, and irritability.

These symptoms of physical hunger could also result from other things. For example, the physical symptoms of hunger are very similar to the physical signs of dehydration. In fact, many people eat when, in fact, their body is craving fluids. So you have to make sure you don't confuse the two.

Separating real hunger from emotional hunger is difficult, especially if you've spent most of your life not listening to your body.

In actuality, a healthy human eater does something very similar to an animal in its natural habitat. A famous Penn State study demonstrated that when children are left to their own devices, they will eat in response to physical cues to hunger. They will stop when they're full. And during any twenty-four-hour period, they will consume a perfectly adequate amount of nutrition.

The problem for the children in this experiment was that when external controls such as when and what they *should* or *should not* eat were placed on them, their biological systems got messed up. Which, by the way, can also happen to animals. Goldfish in captivity, for example, will overeat themselves to death if their well-meaning owner puts too much food in the bowl. Some pet dogs and cats get fat not just because of lack of exercise or because their instinct to hunt is lost in captivity, but also because of how often food is given to them, and the manner in which it is given. When Fido wags his tail and jumps up in anticipation of a "reward" for the trick he has just performed, this exchange between human and dog is about more than merely hunger.

The problem for most compulsive eaters is best described by Mary, who lamented the fact that she never even gets around to asking herself whether she's irritable, or fatigued, or if something else is going on, before she reaches for a fix.

People are the only animals that eat themselves to death.

—AMERICAN MEDICAL ASSOCIATION

PHYSICAL HUNGER CUES

To help you begin to sensitize yourself to how often your eating is in response to *physical* hunger cues, I'd like to offer you a friendly challenge. Don't eat another thing for a while. I can't tell you for how long, because I don't know when or how much you last ate. Drink all the water you want. And see what happens. Does your stomach growl? Do you find yourself getting irritable? Fatigued? Let the physical symptoms emerge. These symptoms will vary from person to person. How our bodies assimilate and use food determines how often we experience them. Typically, though, you will begin to experience the physical cues at three- to four-hour intervals.

When these physical cues of hunger have surfaced, when you really know they're present, eat your meal. This time note how long it takes before the symptoms subside after you have started eating. See how long it takes after you finish your meal before physical symptoms arise again. If you find yourself wanting to reach for food before they have, think about what might be creating this sense of urgency. At the end of this chapter, you'll find a Hunger Awareness Diary. Use it to help you focus on your hunger and eating patterns.

EATING AS A CONDITIONED RESPONSE

Let me ask you a question that may strike you as too personal or too ridiculous or both. How do you know when you have to urinate? The answer is so obvious, you say? You have to go when you have to go. But what tells you that you have to go?

Whether we call it pressure or discomfort, we have physical cues that tell us it's time to go. We don't have to waste a single second thinking about the subject. But what if every hour on the hour you were told to urinate. Day after day. Week after week. What do you think would happen? The answer is that if external controls were placed on you, you'd begin to lose touch with the early physical symptoms, such as pressure on the bladder, that previously appeared spontaneously. You might begin to experience the need to go at the sight of the person who had issued the directive or at the sound of a clock chiming on the hour. Your connection with natural urges would begin to fade and be replaced by what is called a *conditioned response*. If left on your own after this conditioning occurred, it might take more extreme bladder pressure to reconnect you with your body and its basic need.

As Pavlov and his dog so famously demonstrated, the same is true for what goes in as for what goes out. You're probably familiar with this classic experiment, but in a nutshell, what happened was that a dog was conditioned to associate the sound of a bell prior to the arrival of food with the food itself. Ordinarily, the dog would begin to salivate at the sight and smell of the food. After the conditioning, all it took was the bell to elicit the involuntary response of salivation.

This kind of conditioning with regard to human hunger can occur in all sorts of ways. Suppose, for example, that a child comes home from school with an A on a test and shows it to Mom, who is so delighted that she takes a cupcake out of the fridge and serves it with a smile. No doubt a few warm words or a big hug would have done the trick, but with this Mom, food happens to be the way she expresses pleasure in her child.

How long do you think it will take before the child begins to think of food as a reward? Before food becomes associated with having pleased someone? With being loved? With this kind of conditioning, is it possible that the child also begins to think of sweets as a "bribe" to get good grades? That even when studying for a test, the child might have cupcake fantasies?

These kinds of conditioned responses to food can, for some people, play a major role in developing lifelong eating habits. It's called *environmental eating,* which means eating in response to environmental cues.

Eating to me is an inside hug.

—MARY

Fern: "My first association is with popcorn and movies. The second I walk into a movie theater, I head for the refreshment stand. I can remember what it was like as a girl when my mother used to take me to musicals and romantic comedies. It was all so magical, and the popcorn we used to get before the movie began was part of the magic."

Brendan: "Irish soda bread. Just saying the words makes me salivate. My father was into scotch and soda when I was growing up, but I have these great memories of sitting on the kitchen floor while dear old Mom made Irish soda bread and listened to John McCormack records. And I always got the first piece. You want to know how much of an imprint that made? Well, I can tell you that today, if I pass a bakery and get a whiff of Irish soda bread right out of the oven, I'm worse than a bear who's smelled honey. I become a missile that's been fired and is fixed in on its target. A *Playboy* centerfold couldn't distract me from my mission."

Mary: "The first thing that comes to mind—I can't believe I had forgotten about it—is Fig Newtons. I was one of seven kids, and, as you can imagine, my mother had her hands full. There wasn't a whole lot of space given us to be angry or anything. When we were acting up, the first words out of Mom's mouth were 'Wait till your father comes home.' If that didn't work, out came the Fig Newtons. When we got older, we used to call them Mom's 'hush money.' Sometimes, we even *pretended* to be upset just to get Fig Newtons."

Pavlov got his dog to stop salivating at the sound of the bell in the simplest way: He stopped giving the dog food after the ringing of the bell. In other words, he broke the association between the two. After a sufficient number of times in which the bell rang but no food followed, the dog no longer responded to the bell. The salivation response had undergone what is technically called *extinction*.

The two other main methods specialists in behavior-modification techniques use to break through conditioned responses involve introducing *substitute* or *incompatible* behaviors. In the example that Fern cited, we might coach her to enter the movie house with a bag of carrots and a bottle of water as a substitute for the popcorn and soda. If Mary eats her Fig Newtons while she watches television, the behavior-modification specialist might get her to do her knitting there, since you can't eat and knit at the same time.

These kinds of techniques have been found to be helpful in treating the kind of eating that results from conditioned responses to environmental cues. To the extent that some of your eating fits this description, you may benefit from a little behavior modification. However, if the bulk of your eating is in response not to environmental but to psychological cues, these techniques will be ineffective. For compulsive eaters, this is especially true!

PSYCHOLOGICAL HUNGER

Every living thing needs specific forms of stimulation to survive and grow healthily. That includes plants. They need a minimum amount of water. They need nutrients in their soil. Depending on their species, they need so much light and so much warmth. I'm sure all of us know what happens when a houseplant is neglected on any of these counts. Some of you may also recall reading reports that when plants are talked to gently, close up, they really seem to "perk up." Whether they are responding emotionally to the speaker or, more likely, to the carbon dioxide coming from the speaker's mouth, may be open to debate. Either way, they are receiving a welcome form of stimulation.

If plants have basic needs, imagine what we as humans have! When we don't get adequate stimulation, we will inevitably show signs of physical and emotional deterioration. The most terrible example of this

By virtue of being born to humanity, every human being has a right to the development and fulfillment of his potentialities as a human being.

—ASHLEY MONTAGU

can occur with a newborn who gets nothing but an occasional bottle stuck in its mouth. What happens?

What happens is called failure to thrive. The infant just kind of wastes away and dies. We all know that infants need more than regular feeding. They need to be picked up, held, talked to. In the extreme absence of these stimulations, or "strokes" as they are sometimes called, an infant can literally die.

What holds true for infants applies no less to children and adults.

Adults need the same kinds of reinforcement, physically and emotionally. When asked how she felt taken care of, Fern replied, "Just being listened to when you're growing up tells you that you're important."

Brendan said, "How about growing up on a regular diet of kisses and hugs. Or having a dad who's around and sober enough to ask you if you want to have a catch."

Mary added, "If you're a girl and your mother tells you you're really smart or your dad encourages you to play sports, that tells you that you have some value besides being pretty and polite. I had a first-grade teacher who invited me to stay after class and help her pick out books I thought the other kids would like her to read. To this day, my heart— I mean my stomach—just glows when I remember that day more than fifty years ago."

Unfortunately for many of us, the negative messages imprint more strongly. Negative feedback chips away at self-esteem, and most people will fixate on those chips.

Brendan: "It's when you get smacked in the face or hit with a strap. It's when you can't even open your mouth without being punished or told you're a loser. Or when you're constantly hearing things like 'What's the matter with you, can't you do anything right?' "

Fern: "It's your mother always telling you you're too chubby. Or when your father sits at the dinner table and just can't get enough of his son while you sit there feeling invisible."

Mary: "If my mother got upset at us when we were kids, she would first give you a look of anger and disappointment that I can't even describe, and then follow it with the silent treatment. I think an old-fashioned licking would have been easier to take."

During our formative years, the strokes and put-downs we receive from our *external* environment and the way we interpret and react to

Fulfillment is not a true goal to pursue. It is a by-product of our completeness.

—MALCOLM NYGREN

them form the basis of our *inner* emotional environment. Another way of putting it is that we create the plot for our life script. And then, in a way that is at once mysterious and obvious, we grow up and take that script on the road. We turn the world into a movie theater in which we are the projectionist. The audience may change, but somehow we keep showing the same old film.

One of the ways we go about creating this emotional environment or script can be identified just by looking at how we structure our lives in relation to ourselves and others. Throughout the course of the day, we *experience* things and we *interpret* them in ways that more often than not recapitulate the messages we received as young children. And perhaps more striking is the way we keep reliving those negative scenarios.

Mary: "For me, it's like when I stop at the store on the way home from work and buy a quart of ice cream. I tell myself I'm buying it to have around in case any of my kids drops by over the weekend, but by the end of the night I've eaten it all. Then I start putting myself down, telling myself I have no self-discipline, how I'm hopeless."

The self-loathing Mary feels after her rendezvous with Häagen-Dazs is not a new story for her. It is simply Mary's efficient way of using food to play out a scene from her life script. It is a scene from a script Mary knows very intimately because it re-creates the same thoughts and feelings about herself she's had since way back when. The Fig Newtons and ice cream are the vehicles she used to put herself down and create a sense of hopelessness.

It's truly extraordinary how, as we go about re-creating our early emotional world, we gravitate toward certain people and situations that make it easy to complete our mission. And as Mary pointed out, her rendezvous with ice cream demonstrated that *we don't need anyone else to help us.* We can do great "head trips" on ourselves. As a matter of fact, food offers us endless opportunities to connect with our life script in the most interesting ways. Suppose, for example, that you've had a wonderful day, filled with more good news and good contacts with people than you're used to. If all this is too much "stroking" for your script, think of how a good binge before you go to bed will bring you back down to earth.

Why we keep going back to the negative messages is something we'll dwell on in the coming weeks. Let me give you an example now

---

Eating is touch carried to the bitter end.

—SAMUEL BUTLER

of *how* we do it. Suppose I see you in the hall and tell you that you look nice today. How can you turn my compliment into a put-down?

Fern: "I can say to myself that if you think I look nice today, you must think I look terrible all the other days you see me."

Brendan: "I can tell myself you say that to all the guys."

Mary: "Maybe I'll think therapists are *supposed* to say things like that."

You get the idea of how easy it is to negate ourselves? Good.

One thing I would like you to do is follow yourself during this next week and, using the chart below, keep a record of the strokes and put-downs you give yourself. At the end of each day, total up the results. Are you left with more strokes or more put-downs? In other words, how many nights do you go to bed hungry? Psychologically hungry, that is.

Love is the basic need of human nature, for without it, life is disrupted emotionally, mentally, spiritually and physically.

—Dr. Karl Menninger

FOOD FOR THOUGHT

WEEK TWO

Days One Through Seven

• Keep track of your strokes and put-downs each day over the course of this next week by completing the enclosed tally sheet.

• Keep track of your hunger cues each day this week by using the enclosed Hunger Awareness Diary worksheets.

Weekly Checklist

___ 1. Did you complete your Hunger Awareness Diary?

___ 2. Did you complete your Strokes and Put-Downs Tally Sheet?

STROKES AND PUT-DOWNS TALLY SHEET

Instructions: Tally up the strokes and put-downs you receive throughout the day. Highlight or circle those that you receive from *yourself.* Underline those that relate to food, eating, or body weight.

	Strokes	*Put-Downs*
SUNDAY:		
MONDAY:		
TUESDAY:		
WEDNESDAY:		
THURSDAY:		
FRIDAY:		
SATURDAY:		

HUNGER AWARENESS DIARY

Date Time of day	Are you physically hungry? No ——— Yes ——— List your symptoms.	Is your hunger a conditioned response? List environmental cues and triggers.	Are you psychologically hungry? List your thoughts, feelings, cravings.

HUNGER AWARENESS DIARY

Date Time of day	Are you physically hungry? No _____ Yes _____ List your symptoms.	Is your hunger a conditioned response? List environmental cues and triggers.	Are you psychologically hungry? List your thoughts, feelings, cravings.

HUNGER AWARENESS DIARY

Date Time of day	Are you physically hungry? No _____ Yes _____ List your symptoms.	Is your hunger a conditioned response? List environmental cues and triggers.	Are you psychologically hungry? List your thoughts, feelings, cravings.

HUNGER AWARENESS DIARY

Date Time of day	Are you physically hungry? No ——— Yes ——— List your symptoms.	Is your hunger a conditioned response? List environmental cues and triggers.	Are you psychologically hungry? List your thoughts, feelings, cravings.

HUNGER AWARENESS DIARY

Date Time of day	Are you physically hungry? No ___ Yes ___ List your symptoms.	Is your hunger a conditioned response? List environmental cues and triggers.	Are you psychologically hungry? List your thoughts, feelings, cravings.

HUNGER AWARENESS DIARY

Date Time of day	Are you physically hungry? No ____ Yes ____ List your symptoms.	Is your hunger a conditioned response? List environmental cues and triggers.	Are you psychologically hungry? List your thoughts, feelings, cravings.

HUNGER AWARENESS DIARY

Date Time of day	Are you physically hungry? No _____ Yes _____ List your symptoms.	Is your hunger a conditioned response? List environmental cues and triggers.	Are you psychologically hungry? List your thoughts, feelings, cravings.

Family Ties

~

This week you will attend a family reunion. During the visit you will do some digging to uncover your compulsive-eating roots.

Family reunions stir up lots of feelings, not all of them pleasant, especially if you struggle with your weight. The first thing you probably think is, "I've got to lose weight before going home." It's understandable, then, that you may not be in a hurry to sign up for this trip. Generous soul that I am, let me offer you a few minutes' delay in flight-departure time.

How did last week's homework go? Let's start with the Hunger Awareness Diary. First of all, did you do it? Brendan didn't.

Brendan: "I know what you're going to say, but I had a hellish week. Didn't have a second to myself. I promise. Next week."

If you did keep a diary, even for one day, was it helpful?

Fern: "I'm not sure. I felt a little like I did eating in front of the mirror. I mean, very self-conscious. Especially at night. So I was always asking myself if I was physically hungry, and of course most of the time I wasn't, and that made it hard for me to eat the way I usually do. The only feeling I remember having was anger. Mainly at you for making me do this."

Mary: "I kept the diary, and as for Fern, it confirmed what is becoming pretty clear to all of us—that my compulsive eating is really about feelings. I must admit that I didn't let those feelings stick around long before I put something in my mouth, but what I do remember welling up in me was sadness. This overwhelming feeling of sadness." (As Mary recounted this, her eyes filled with tears and she cried quietly.)

If you experienced thoughts and feelings doing your diary, remember them. They're yours, and they're important.

Now, how about the strokes and put-downs? What did you receive? What did you give yourself?

Fern: "Mostly put-downs and mostly about being out of control with my eating. The best or worst example, depending on how you look at it, was Saturday night. Around ten o'clock, I went down to the deli. I told myself I needed milk—and managed to come home with a box of doughnuts. I ate five in a couple of minutes. I was so disgusted with myself that on Sunday I didn't leave my apartment and I didn't answer my phone."

Brendan: "As I said, I was too busy to really focus on this, but my major put-down for the week has been today, when I learned I had gained weight. What does that tell me about myself? The words that come to mind I do not use in front of ladies."

Mary: "I put myself down for all kinds of things. Not being a good enough nurse or wife or whatever. But mostly, my negative feelings were like Brendan's and Fern's. I beat myself up mostly around food and eating issues."

How did you do with the exercise? Did you keep a list? What did your tally sheet look like? How many times did you turn a possible stroke into a put-down? Any idea why? To answer my last question brings us directly into this week: Family Ties.

By now you've probably figured out that I have a thing about animals. I may be especially partial to lionesses, perhaps because they carry the burden of hunting and cub-raising, but you don't hear anyone referring to them as "Queen of the Beasts." Oh, well. When lion cubs grow up and leave home or join the pride, they undoubtedly carry with them a few "messages" necessary for their survival. They have learned by observation and experience how to find and catch food. They have developed the knowledge they need to stay out of the way of poisonous snakes. We also know that, *The Lion King* notwithstanding, in real life the male is an absentee father. And Mom? Does she

I am a turtle. Wherever I go I carry "home" on my back.

—GLORIA ANZALDUA

give her kids any messages about food or their weight? Does she hand out any strokes or put-downs in general? If there were such a thing as lion therapy, would we hear a young lion say that he felt his father was distant and never loved him? Would a lioness remember how her mother had berated her for being overweight?

Not likely, although some would note that animals do indeed react profoundly to such traumatic events as being orphaned. If you have ever encountered a dog that has been abused, you can see it in the way it carries itself, its mistrust of people, and how it responds to loving care.

We humans, on the other hand, send and receive all kinds of complex messages to each other. And nowhere are these messages more important, is the imprinting greater, than those that occur between parents and children. "Nearly all human activity is programmed by an ongoing script dating from early childhood" is the way the psychiatrist Eric Berne, M.D., put it. And no small wonder. First impressions, as they say, can be lasting. You'd be surprised at how many earlies or firsts we retain. Use the space below to write down some of the pleasurable first moments you remember. Riding a bike on your own? Your first movie? Something you did with a relative? Close your eyes and see where you go.

First Memory #1: _____
_____

First Memory #2: _____
_____

First Memory #3: _____
_____

Fern: "What immediately came to mind was my father swinging me in a hammock. I must have been two or three at the most. I remember the hammock was green and it was strung between two white birch trees next to a summer cottage my parents had rented. It must have been my first time in a hammock, and I think I was a little scared at first, but I remember my father gently rocking it and singing 'Summertime,' and the next thing I knew I was asleep."

Family quarrels are bitter things. They don't go according to any rules. They're not like aches or wounds. They're more like splits in the skin that won't heal because there's not enough material.

—F. SCOTT FITZGERALD

Brendan: "I certainly remember the first time I had sex. Unfortunately, it was so exciting that the memory is a very fleeting one, if you get my drift."

Mary: "Maybe it's because we're here, but my first memories to surface are food ones and they all have to do with my grandmother, who lived with us. When I would come home from school, she would always be waiting with freshly baked cookies or brownies or whatever. Now, whether my brothers and sisters were around or I brought home friends, she always seemed to make sure I got the biggest one. I really think I was her favorite. I mean, I know this is complicated because I have food issues, but back then there was nothing complicated about it. It made me feel terrific. Now I do the same thing for special people."

Whether it was Fern's specific memory, Brendan's "fleeting" or Mary's collective one, you probably get the sense that they are all deeply stored and not insignificant. How about the ones you retrieved? Spend a few moments now thinking about why they are emotionally important for you.

EARLY DECISIONS

You don't need me to tell you that beyond specific moments, family members constantly cross-fertilize each other with attitudes and behavior. Food and eating are just one arena where love and affection are demonstrated or withheld. Where anger is displayed or hidden. How individuality is encouraged or frowned on. Whether cooperation or competition rules the day. Or how success is defined. The family is where we first get the message that acceptance is based on performance or not. Similar or different messages are sent to boys and girls regarding attitudes about sexuality, looks, and whether the world outside our home is basically friendly or hostile.

The list could go on and on, but the underlying point is that the messages we are given from significant people in our lives—parents, siblings, grandparents, nannies, teachers, friends—carry with them detailed inscriptions creating in us character traits that form the basis of decisions we make about ourselves. This process results in what is commonly called our self-image, including that oft-used expression, our *self-esteem.*

Happy or unhappy families are all mysterious. We have only to imagine how differently we would be described—and will be after our deaths—by each of the family members who believe they know us.

—GLORIA STEINEM

These early decisions we make about ourselves, which are based on not only the messages we receive but the way we react to them, set the stage for the way we will experience ourselves in relation to ourselves and therefore to the world. This life script with which we emerge from childhood contains a mosaic of complex feelings that will affect our emotional "take" on almost everything. If we never stop to examine this, if we become the human equivalents of the automatic cruise-control device some cars are equipped with, then we will continue to follow the same old route over and over. And like a driver who nods off with the cruise control on, we will continue to crash in the same old way.

The method in which our scripts are written works wonderfully, of course, for people who grew up in a secure and loving environment. Their needs were, for the most part, identified and met. The nurturing they received allowed them to blossom with a sense of love, security, autonomy, and trust. They learned how to soothe, comfort, and pleasure themselves, and at the same time set appropriate limits for themselves and others. They operate much like baleen whales, who are graced with marvelous equipment that allows them to suck in everything around them, take in what's nourishing, and filter out the rest.

If this sounds a little like a Walt Disney fantasy, if you're waiting to hear the bluebirds of happiness chirping in the background, you're right. If we grow up in a gardenlike environment, it is never the Garden of Eden. Human perfection is an oxymoron. Since to err is human, it not only can happen, it will happen. Besides, a "perfect" childhood, whatever that might be, would actually be a disaster if you consider that our life's task is to grow up and leave home. After all, no one would voluntarily leave the Garden of Eden.

So perfection is not what I'm talking about. The question is whether the environment you grew up in was good enough to flourish in. Children who grow up in negative or emotionally confusing environments, who don't receive enough intimacy, nurturing, and love in ways that imprint on them, will invariably emerge with a very different sense of themselves. They will often be left with a deep, aching emptiness. They will yearn for intimacy and at the same time run from it. They will typically experience feelings of powerlessness, guilt, anger, sadness, isolation (Brendan: "It's what I call my black hole"). They will feel unloved and, worse, unlovable.

It is a wise father that knows his own child.

—WILLIAM SHAKESPEARE

Again, let's not paint this as an either/or scenario. That would be too simplistic. If we got nothing but negative messages growing up, we wouldn't be here to talk about it. Believe it or not, the mere fact that you've gotten this far in *The Hunger Within* is proof that you have many strengths! Without them, you could not even allow yourself to hope that maybe, however remote the possibility, something about your compulsive eating might change.

When the "well" in our sense of well-being feels empty, we seek to fill it. When we can't draw on the real thing for nourishment, we seek substitutes. Workaholism, various forms of substance abuse, compulsive behavior, masochistic relationships—these are just a few of the options available to us. Oh, yes. And then there's food.

Let's focus now on some of the early messages we got about eating that may reveal something about our *emotional* relationship with it. Take a moment and see if you can think of anything that might explain why you use food to fill your empty well: _____

_____

_____

_____

All happy families resemble one another, but each unhappy family is unhappy in its own way.

—LEO TOLSTOY

Fern: "When I think of my mother, the first word I'd use to describe what I feel and always felt is 'unsafe.' I felt unsafe around food because my mother was so controlling about it. She was the mother, she put food on the table, and she was a micromanager of our meals. She monitored what every person ate. Still does. When I was growing up, she would serve all of us meat and a vegetable, and then give potatoes only to Daddy and my brother. None of us were fat or really overweight. It didn't matter. She never asked me 'Do you want a potato?' any more than she asked my brother if he didn't. He even makes jokes about it now when we visit her, but he never got fat. I think her control drove him crazy, too, but he wouldn't be manipulated by her, at least with food. I don't know if that's because he was the boy in the family, or because he got the potato. I do know that my mother was always talking about women having to watch their weight. So did her mother. I think they thought that was the way you got a man and kept him. Well, she couldn't keep my father, because he died when I was a teenager. And I must be a hell of a rebel, because here I am in my thirties, fat and single, a living testament to my mother's failure to control me."

Brendan: "Something that Fern said about control rang a Pavlovian

$\mathcal{H}$e that loves not his
wife and children feeds a
lioness at home and
broods a nest of sorrows.

— JEREMY TAYLOR

bell for me. I talked last week about my mother's Irish soda bread and how much I loved it and still do. So the obvious connection is that I associate food with love. But come to think of it, maybe my mother also used food to control me. If I haven't made it clear by now, I grew up in an alcoholic home. My father was a mean drunk. Verbally and physically. For whatever reasons, my mother wasn't about to leave him, so, needless to say, it was hardly a serene environment when you didn't know when the front door opened whether a monster was walking in or you had a temporary reprieve. In that situation, there wasn't a whole lot of space for any of the rest of us to be angry or anything else negative. Dear old Dad had a monopoly on that. I think my mother, the saint, needed us kids to be angels. And I have this feeling that she used food to placate us or sedate us or something. Of all the terrible memories I have, maybe the worst was the night my father went after my mother and slapped her. I was only ten or eleven, but I jumped between them to try to stop him. My father picked me up and threw me across the room. I was practically unconscious. Now get this: I'm lying there and my father stops hitting my mother and he starts sobbing about what a bastard he is and who do you think my mother comforts? Him!

"But the story doesn't end there. My mother goes off to help my father to bed, and a few minutes later she comes back and takes me by the hand and leads me into the kitchen and starts feeding me cookies and who knows what. So was that love? Or was the idea that if I ate I wouldn't be upset or anything else she couldn't handle? It wasn't just that time either. I think she regularly would offer food whenever any of us displayed strong emotions, especially anger. She must have done that with herself, too, because she's not exactly a skinny Minnie."

Family therapists frequently use something called a *genogram* to help them get beyond the specific problems being talked about so they can help identify and address the underlying emotional themes that may be creating difficulties. Basically a genogram is a kind of family map, or tree, in which at least three generations of the family and extended family are represented visually. We can then ask questions about almost any subject to see whether a pattern emerges. Have marriages been good or bad? Is there a history of alcoholism or substance abuse? Physical or mental illness? Violence? Money problems? Favored offspring?

I always ask my group to play detective and do their own genograms. The first and most basic goal is to track the history of compulsive eating, obesity, messages about food that were passed down. Beyond that, we want to learn who had good or bad, close or distant relationships. Who was available to be nurturing. Who was not and why.

When we've put down everything, we'll step back to see what kinds of clues we can come up with that might help us understand how and why we came to be compulsive eaters.

What follows is the genogram Fern came up with for her family. Study it carefully before you move on to read Fern's reaction.

As is the mother, so is her daughter.

—EZEKIEL 16:44

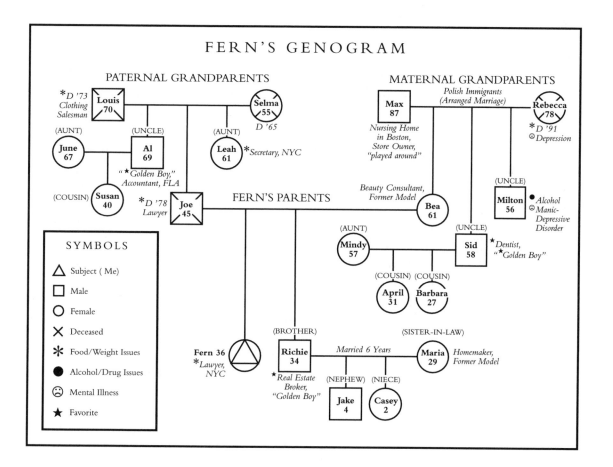

FERN'S GENOGRAM

Fern: "The first thing I realized looking at my genogram was not a 'food' thing. It was that my family has so many 'favorite sons' we could have a political convention. My father's older brother, Al, was his parents' favorite. My mother's younger brother, Sid, was the golden boy in that family. And in my family, it was my brother, Richie, who could do no wrong. I think it's interesting that both my parents were *not* the preferred sibling, and then they do the same thing with their kids. I think it's sick. Why should there be favorites? You'd think if you decide to have kids, you'd love them all equally.

"As far as the family dynamics about food, my father had food issues just like his father. I don't know where Grandpa Louis got his from, but I remember that even though Uncle Al was the favorite, he apparently was a lousy eater. Grandma Selma used to cook all the time, and I think she used to praise my father for being a *good* eater. So maybe this was his main opportunity to shine and he just kept eating because it made him feel emotionally that he was getting his mother's blessing. What's weird is that when he married my mother, he got a completely different reaction to his eating. Maybe that was when he started to eat secretly. It must all have been very confusing for him.

"Then there was my mother, who had food issues because of the way she controlled what I ate, but she wasn't a compulsive eater herself. What dawns on me now, looking at my genogram, is why she made such a big deal of it. I knew she had been a model when she was young, but to tell you the truth, I've never thought much more about it. What's occurring to me now is that my mother's mother, Grandma Rebecca, was fat and my Grandpa Max played around. It was an arranged marriage without much love that I could tell. I think Grandpa Max made very little effort to hide the fact that he had something going with some of the younger women who came into his lingerie store downtown. So maybe my mother grew up thinking that if she stayed thin, her father would love *her*. Or that when she grew up, this was the way to keep a man. If this was the case, if she meant well by passing this message on to me by shoving it down my throat, it sure didn't help.

"If I'm right, then my father ate to be loved and my mother didn't eat to be loved. This is making me dizzy."

No small wonder. Fern will make some vitally important new connections for herself when she revisits her genogram next week, but for now let's turn for a few minutes to Brendan and Mary.

Men are what their mothers made them.

—RALPH WALDO EMERSON

Brendan: "For me, the main things to jump off the page were my father being an alcoholic and my mother having her hands full with him and how, as I'm starting to realize, she may have used food to sedate us kids, particularly me and one of my sisters. The two of us were considered the 'troublemakers,' although in another family we might have been considered pretty good.

"What's obvious to me is that my mother needed me to go along with the program, and food was the way to keep me quiet. So maybe that's what I do now—use food to sit on my feelings because as a kid I 'decided,' to use your expression, that nobody was there for me and that what I felt didn't matter. Of course, I've done this so long that I wouldn't even have a clue what feelings I might be sitting on, assuming I have any in the first place. I guess I also learned that it's safer to have a relationship with food than with people. I don't really let anyone get that close to me or vice versa. I think I use humor a lot for that. But I'll tell you one way I just realized that my past works for me. In my career. Being a stockbroker is just like being in the house I grew up in. Every day, you can't predict if the market's going up or down. And if it goes down, there are always plenty of people to blame you. At least when people make money with me, I get paid well *and* I get praised. That's something I didn't get at home."

Mary: "In some ways, I have quite a bit in common with Brendan. My parents weren't really available either. My father worked a whole lot because he had to with a wife and seven kids or because it was easier to work than be at home. Either way, he wasn't very affectionate, physically or emotionally. And my mom, she wasn't just overwhelmed by all those kids, but she had these episodes—they used to call them 'nervous breakdowns'—today they'd be diagnosed as depression. So she was hospitalized several times and you couldn't really expect much from her.

"I was the oldest girl, and even though my grandmother was around most of the time, it was really my job to baby-sit the little ones. I think I had to grow up very fast. I don't think I had much of a childhood. Certainly, I must have learned that everyone else's needs were more important than mine. Maybe that I didn't deserve to have my needs met. I sure have been playing the role of caretaker my whole life. As a kid. As a wife and mother. Now as a nurse. I suppose I'm hoping that if I give enough, someone will take care of me. That I won't always be waiting for my grandmother's cookie. But the thing is, I don't even

There are no conditions to which a man cannot become accustomed, especially if he sees that all those around him live the same way.

—LEO TOLSTOY

state my needs. So I can't blame anyone but myself if they're not met. Right?"

Mary raises a profoundly important point when she recognizes that she keeps her needs to herself. It's one we'll be getting back to in many ways. For now, however, I'd like to end this chapter by getting back to you.

Sometime in the next few days—there would be no better time than now if it's possible—I want you to fill in the genogram outlined at the end of the chapter. Don't be intimidated if you can't remember every relative or if you don't know whether they had any issues with food or compulsions. Fill it in as best you can.

Based on the discussions you've heard this week, see what you can learn about the history and meaning of food in *your* family. What other themes emerge that might bear directly on the script you wrote for yourself as a child? If you can, keep notes on how these themes continue to play themselves out in your life on a daily basis. The more you write, the more likely you'll see patterns emerge that keep you from your most desired goal: *change.*

We often get in quicker by the back door than by the front.

—NAPOLEON I

FOOD FOR THOUGHT

WEEK THREE

Day One

Complete the following chart:

Name of mother	Messages I received	Decisions, conclusions, and beliefs I made about myself based on these messages

Day Two

Complete the following chart:

Name of father	Messages I received	Decisions, conclusions, and beliefs I made about myself based on these messages

Day Three

Complete the following chart:

Name of grandparents	Messages I received	Decisions, conclusions, and beliefs I made about myself based on these messages

Day Four

Complete the following chart:

Name of siblings	Messages I received	Decisions, conclusions, and beliefs I made about myself based on these messages

Day Five

Draw out or fill in the seating arrangement at your family dinner table when you were a child.

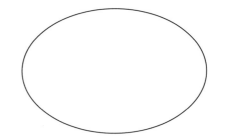

Reflect on how you felt in your designated seat:_____

_____

Day Six

Try to recall what your family dinners were like: Who was there? ____

_____

What was served? _____

What was discussed? _____

How were you feeling?_____

Day Seven

Draw your dinner table today.

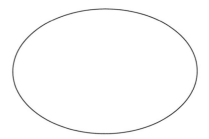

Fill in where you and any other members of your family would typically be seated. Describe: _____

_____

Weekly Checklist

___ 1. Did you complete your genogram? Use the My Genogram Worksheet, located at the end of this chapter.

___ 2. Did you complete your Food for Thought exercises?

___ 3. Are you still keeping track of strokes and put-downs? See enclosed tally sheet.

___ 4. Have you been able to leave a little food on your plate at the end of a meal?

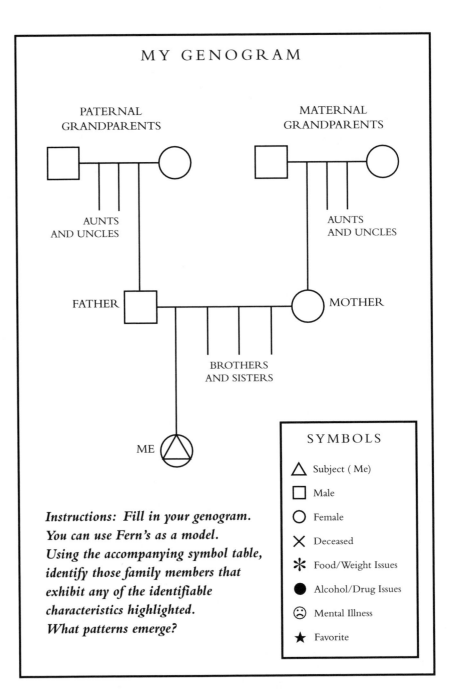

MY GENOGRAM

PATERNAL
GRANDPARENTS

MATERNAL
GRANDPARENTS

AUNTS
AND UNCLES

AUNTS
AND UNCLES

FATHER

MOTHER

BROTHERS
AND SISTERS

ME

*Instructions: Fill in your genogram.
You can use Fern's as a model.
Using the accompanying symbol table,
identify those family members that
exhibit any of the identifiable
characteristics highlighted.
What patterns emerge?*

SYMBOLS

△ Subject (Me)

□ Male

○ Female

✕ Deceased

✳ Food/Weight Issues

● Alcohol/Drug Issues

☹ Mental Illness

★ Favorite

STROKES AND PUT-DOWNS TALLY SHEET

Instructions: Tally up the strokes and put-downs you receive throughout the day. Highlight or circle those that you receive from *yourself.* Underline those that relate to food, eating, or body weight.

	Strokes	Put-Downs
SUNDAY:		
MONDAY:		
TUESDAY:		
WEDNESDAY:		
THURSDAY:		
FRIDAY:		
SATURDAY:		

The Scariest Word

❧

When you repress or suppress the things which you don't want to live with, you don't really solve the problem because you don't bury the problem dead—you bury it alive and active within you.

—JOHN POWELL

This week you will come face to face with the great white shark of living: change. And we'll pay our respects to the part of you that wants to stay out of the water!

Before you begin this chapter, please fill in your genogram if you haven't done so already. It will really help you lay the groundwork for the material we're going to cover this week, as we draw to the end of Stage One, and in the weeks to come. You may, for example, have a belated response to your genogram, as Fern did, which none of us could have anticipated. For Fern, it was a realization that went to the core of her being and was the key that opened the door to the mystery of her compulsive eating. And paradoxically, of course, it had everything to do with food and nothing to do with food. We'll get to Fern's story, but for now close your eyes for a few moments and let the word "change" cross your mind like a banner trailing a small plane that passes by while you're lying on the beach. Let the word stir up whatever it does. Let yourself free-associate and jot down the images that come to mind:

_____

_____

_____

_____

Fern: "When my eyes were closed, I actually got a sinking feeling in my stomach and the first associations I had were how upsetting it used to be for me every year the day before I left for sleepaway camp or the first day of school. Believe it or not, I couldn't eat at those times. I was too anxious. And the weird thing is, I really looked forward to school and camp. In fact, I loved them."

Brendan: "I had exactly the opposite reaction to Fern's. What came into my mind was an image of myself standing chest deep in turquoise water off a beautiful beach in the Caribbean. I was filled with a great sense of well-being. It was late afternoon. The sun was soft. I could almost feel my skin changing from sickly white to golden tan. That's where the word 'change' took me, perhaps because you introduced the beach image with the banner trailing, but for whatever reason, all I could think of was how nice a change would be."

Mary: "I did not like where the word 'change' took me. When I free-associated with that word, what came into my mind was 'changing room' like in a department store. I kept getting images of trying on things and nothing fit and it was all very unpleasant. The next thing I thought of was 'small change,' like in money. That was actually better. The word 'small' seemed very comforting, but I don't know if that related to body size or that change is so scary because it seems like such a big deal."

When it comes to the word "change," Mary hit the proverbial nail on the head. For most of us, the prospect of change means leaving what we know, however miserable that might be, for the great unknown. Perhaps that's why we're so awestruck by accounts of the early explorers. Symbolically, they represent all that we, sitting on our couch and munching potato chips, might feel about the prospect of entering uncharted waters. There is a part of all of us that fantasizes regularly about how wonderful change would be. If we won the lottery. Lived somewhere spectacular. Went on an incredible vacation. Dare I say it, were no longer overweight or controlled by our food compulsion.

Change is a little like becoming intimate with someone who really turns us on. The wave of desire urges us to plunge in, even though we don't know if it's going to turn out well or whether we'll drown.

During our group session I like to lead our participants in a communal visualization exercise to illustrate the dilemma. Close your eyes

Things do not change. We do.

—HENRY DAVID THOREAU

again. This time imagine a country lake, frozen in winter beauty. Imagine yourself standing on a darkened shore in early evening. Out in the middle of the lake, a group of people have lit up an area with lanterns. Some are skating, others are dancing under a full moon.

You, on the other hand, are standing alone on the darkened shore. As the sounds of merriment float seductively toward you, a deep longing surges to be out there where the fun is. What do you do? Keep your eyes closed and watch yourself enter the scene.

Fern: "It may seem overly cautious—which is what makes me a good lawyer, by the way—but I'm not at all sure what I'd do in this situation. After all, I don't know who these people are. I don't mean that I think they might be killers, but it could be a family or club outing and they might make it clear that strangers were not welcome. Going out there and getting a chilly reception would be worse for me than not going out. On the other hand, I realize the possible advantages of taking a risk."

Brendan: "This one is a no-brainer for me. I'm on the way out there! If there's anything I know how to do, it's 'schmooze.' It may be their party, but I guarantee you that by the time it's over, I'll be the life of it. I don't mean to brag, but this is one area where I know myself."

Mary: "I guess it's pretty clear by now that at least superficially, Brendan and I are very different. In this case, I know myself also, and I know I would *not* go. It wouldn't even *occur* to me to go. Probably because I'm so shy. For Fern, it sounds like she'd have to make a decision. I wouldn't."

Something is going on out on the frozen lake that could be wonderful, but only Brendan clearly wants to make a move. Perhaps that's because Brendan tells us there's no risk involved for him; he's confident he'll succeed.

For Fern and Mary, the possibilities are more treacherous. Doubt and fear dog their ability to enter the scene. What if the ice is thick in some parts but treacherously thin in others? How do you know if you "go for it" that you won't fall through?

Taking risks and changing involves a certain level of uncertainty, which is one reason people resist it. As uncomfortable as we may be with our lives, simply staying within our self-imposed limits provides a level of emotional safety. We may long for the fun and intrigue that may await us in the middle of the lake, but we are on intimate terms with the protected part of ourselves safely here on shore.

But there's more. Who we are, among other things, is the sum total of defenses we unconsciously developed as children to protect ourselves. These defenses have technical names like *denial, isolation, intellectualization, projection, displacement, undoing,* and *regression.* I like to think of them, however, as the Seven Dwarfs. Defense mechanisms may sound like something bad. Quite the opposite. At least when we first created them, they were adaptive. They were our friends. We used them to help protect us from the Evil Queen. At stake was nothing less than our survival.

Here are a few examples to show you what I mean. When an older sibling who is already toilet-trained begins soiling himself soon after the arrival of a new baby in the house, the *regression* is adaptive. Why? This change in the family system created a level of vulnerability in the older sibling that caused him to regress back to past, familiar patterns in attempts to recapture the world he knew prior to the birth of the new baby. It may also be a forceful reminder to the parents that there is another child in the household who still needs attention.

Likewise, we can do this same thing with our eating patterns and our body weight. Often when we encounter a change—a new job, getting married, a move to a new location—we will find ourselves *regressing* back to our old patterns, an adaptation we use in attempts to bring us back to what we know.

One more illustration: A person experiences the traumatic loss of a loved one. Although she is told this person has died, she continues to act as though the loved one is still there, talking to the deceased, even making gifts to give to the person at Christmas. We would say this person is in *denial,* but surely we can appreciate how this defense mechanism helps, at least in a transitional sense, the absorption of unfathomable grief.

How about you? What defense mechanisms did you develop to survive? Why were they needed? Do you still use them now that you are an adult? How?

Fern: "I'll plead to *displacement* and *isolation.* I don't like myself for it, but there are plenty of times that I'm furious at something, like my encounter with the car dealer, but I don't confront the person. Then later, I find myself turning my anger against myself by bingeing to stuff down my feelings and later beating myself up. In that situation I then

True life is lived when tiny changes occur.

—LEO TOLSTOY

went on to *isolate* myself, immersed in guilt and self-disgust, by staying in my apartment and refusing to answer the phone. I realized it afterward, but I still keep doing it."

Brendan: "I'm big into denial. I'd like to deny that this is the case, but I can't. I denied for years that I was an alcoholic. I still look into the mirror and see a thin man with a full head of hair. I guess when I make jokes about my doctor's warnings to me and disregard his advice, that's another form of denial. I think *projection* is also my thing. I've started to realize that sometimes I feel someone else is angry at me, when the reverse is actually true. I'm angry at myself. I find that I *project* a lot of my thoughts and feelings onto others."

Mary: "Denial is one I sure use a lot also, but my favorite is probably *undoing.* I understand that means that when you feel guilty for something you think or feel or do, you do something to atone for it or make it go away. I probably became an expert in this after years of going to confession in church, but I do it in lots of other ways. For example, every time I go off into one of my eating frenzies I find myself feeling so guilty that the next day I will fast to undo the 'damage' that I created. I know I also do a lot of *rationalizing* or *intellectualizing* or whatever they call it. I know when I was a kid I was always giving myself reasons why my dad had no time for me, or my mom either, for that matter. What good would it have done for me to have protested?"

To change, to move into unfamiliar territory, means letting down our defenses. And at what cost? The possibility of falling through the ice? No wonder we're cautious!

Let me give you an example of what I mean that relates directly to why you bought this book in the first place: your eating and your weight. On the following page is an exercise I call Body Size/Feeling State. What I'd like you to do now is use the worksheet and list all the things you can think of that describe who the *thin* you is/was/would be and who the *fat* you is/was/would be in each of the four categories listed. Use one or two words for each description, and write down anything that comes to mind.

Let me assert my firm belief that the only thing we have to fear is fear itself.

—FRANKLIN D. ROOSEVELT

BODY SIZE/FEELING STATE EXERCISE

Instructions: Select the appropriate adjective to describe yourself when completing the statements below. Using pictures or words, describe how you would feel professionally, socially, emotionally, and physically in each body state.

The "fat" me is . . . was . . . would be . . .

Physically	Emotionally	Professionally	Socially

The "thin" me is . . . was . . . would be . . .

Physically	Emotionally	Professionally	Socially

Here are some of the things Fern, Brendan, and Mary wrote:

FERN: The fat me is: physically crippled
                                       emotionally sedated
                                       professionally limited
                                       socially distanced

               The thin me would be: physically sexy
                                       emotionally more vulnerable
                                       professionally challenged
                                       socially more competitive

BRENDAN: The fat me is: physically inert
                                       emotionally safe
                                       professionally accommodating
                                       socially popular

               The thin me would be: physically more energetic
                                       emotionally more serious
                                       professionally more secure
                                       socially more intimate

MARY: The fat me is: physically unhealthy
                                       emotionally depressed
                                       professionally walked over
                                       socially invisible

               The thin me would be: physically attractive/active
                                       emotionally confused
                                       professionally respected
                                       socially more in
                                       demand/demanding

❧

Our doubts are traitors,
And make us lose the
good we oft might win,
By fearing to attempt.

—WILLIAM SHAKESPEARE

In filling out this chart it should become clear whether you are a creature of habit, if you simply find comfort in the familiarity of everything, including your weight, or whether the prospect of change brings out one or more of your defensive dwarfs for more complex reasons. If your responses were honest, they should probably signal how mired and invested you are in staying safe behind a wall of food.

Fern: "When I look at what I wrote, I can see how one could make the case that I use my weight defensively. I did say that the thin me would be physically sexy and emotionally more vulnerable. Without going into too much detail, I'll say that being sexy and vulnerable are not necessarily positive things for me."

Brendan: "I'm not sure what defenses I use by being fat, but I'm on the same page as Fern with this. Three of the four things on my 'thin' me list—physically more energetic, emotionally more serious, and socially more intimate—these three may sound wonderful but actually the words make me more anxious than joyful. Only being professionally more secure doesn't give my blood pressure a little jolt."

Mary: "I can see that it is the same for me. This is difficult for me to admit, but I am sure that I have used my body weight to create a barrier between myself and my husband. In fact [Mary stutters in hesitation], what brought me to this workshop is the fact that my husband has been getting home late over the last few months. Six weeks ago I actually found a woman's name and telephone number on a piece of paper tucked into the back pocket of his trousers while I was doing the laundry. I was so upset that the first thing I did was *eat*. I must admit that it was that particular incident that brought me into this program one month ago, and am I glad it did."

As Fern, Brendan, and Mary began to realize by doing this exercise, our body weight can definitely be used as a suit of armor that protects us from others. When our early environments were not safe and did not allow us to have effective boundaries, increased body weight can become an imaginary boundary. It can be used as a defense mechanism that allows us to distance ourselves from the real or anticipated danger of being close to others. Even more, it can protect us from our unconscious fear of something even scarier: getting close to ourselves.

Do Fern, Brendan, and Mary speak to you? How might it be dangerous for you to be thin? Try to sift through the emotions of it until you unearth some connections that might help you understand how you use body weight defensively and why changing your body size might be so understandably frightening.

Food and eating, as we identified in Week One, serve a *function* for us. Likewise, our body size serves a *function* for us as well. What defense mechanism might be operating for us in reference to food, eating, and body weight?

All changes, even the most longed for, have their melancholy; for what we leave behind us is a part of ourselves; we must die to one life before we can enter into another.

—ANATOLE FRANCE

*I reject get-it-done,
make-it-happen thinking.
I want to slow things
down so I understand
them better.*

— JERRY BROWN

Fern had a belated response to her genogram that helped her to answer this very question. It was an awareness that profoundly affected her. "I left here last week thinking about food in my family," she said. "I've talked before about how my mother controlled the way food was doled out and how important it was for her that the women be slim, maybe because her mom was heavy and her dad fooled around. I talked to my brother about all this and he said he wasn't sure, but he wouldn't be surprised if Mom was bulimic when she was a model. He said that a few years ago, he was having dinner with Mom and she was talking about my weight and how upsetting it was for her. He said he asked her whether she had any weight issues herself when she was younger and she said she had. And when he asked her what she had done to help herself, she had said, 'You do what you have to do.' Then she made it clear the conversation was over. He wasn't sure how much more he wanted to hear anyway."

Doing the genogram started the ball rolling for Fern. She learned about her mother's relationship with food, which may have been passed down to her in a different form. But the family secret Fern had been obsessing about had nothing to do with her mother.

Fern: "I can't believe I haven't made this connection before. You see, I know my father had food issues himself. I've always known that. Sometimes late at night he and I would meet in the kitchen looking for food that my mom had not served or served enough of. He even had a little hiding place where he kept candy he brought home.

"It was like some childhood game we shared together. We would stand there in the dark and gobble down stuff, being 'bad' together and checking to make sure Mommy didn't catch us. I'm not sure, but I think we were doing that the night before he died. And that's what came back to me this week, this one thing he and I had that was so special, that not even my brother had with him."

Special? How does one begin to describe special? Or what Fern's "compulsive" eating might mean in light of this memory? And most important, why Fern, regardless of how inviting it might seem to lose weight and say good-bye to being out of control with food, might not be in such a hurry to embrace change that might also mean saying good-bye to her father.

We'll be getting back to Fern, her dad, and the implications of change in the weeks to come. For now, as we conclude this week, I'd like to urge you to continue to search for the special connections you have with your own family and food. The more you uncover, the better equipped you'll be to consider your options.

FOOD FOR THOUGHT

WEEK FOUR

Day One

Stand on the scale and look at the number for not less than thirty seconds. Get off and write down the number. Look at it.
What does this number represent to you? _____

_____

Day Two

Close your eyes and stand on the scale. Fantasize that the scale reads twenty pounds less than yesterday.
When do you remember weighing this amount?_____
Describe:_____

_____
What thoughts and feelings does this number elicit? _____

_____

There is a time for departure even when there's no certain place to go.

—TENNESSEE WILLIAMS

Day Three

Stand on the scale and imagine the numbers going down before your eyes. At what number do you begin to feel anxious?
Write down everything that comes to mind about this number. ____

_____

Day Four

Cover the scale with tape. Get on. With no access to a number, record how you feel about yourself. _____

_____

Day Five

Do not get on the scale today. What messages are you telling yourself about your body? _____
_____

Day Six

Imagine your weight being broadcast in Times Square, or a nurse shouting it out so a waiting room full of patients can hear it. Describe your feelings:_____
_____

*The moment of change
is the only poem.*

—ADRIENNE RICH

Day Seven

Get back on the scale and record your actual weight. Is it up or down from the beginning of the week? How does the change affect how you feel about yourself? _____
_____

Weekly Checklist

____ 1. Did you complete the Body Size/Feeling State exercise?

____ 2. Did you complete your Food for Thought writing exercises?

____ 3. Are you still keeping track of strokes and put-downs? See enclosed tally sheet.

____ 4. Have you been able to leave a little food on your plate at the end of a meal?

STROKES AND PUT-DOWNS TALLY SHEET

Instructions: Tally up the strokes and put-downs you receive throughout the day. Highlight or circle those that you receive from *yourself*. Underline those that relate to food, eating, or body weight.

	Strokes	*Put-Downs*
SUNDAY:		
MONDAY:		
TUESDAY:		
WEDNESDAY:		
THURSDAY:		
FRIDAY:		
SATURDAY:		

Stage Two

❧

Discovery

The Vicious Cycle

❧

Ever find yourself driving around for an hour and accidentally ending up where you started? This week you'll learn that when you do it in your personal life, it's no accident.

I want to begin this week by having a little fun. What I'd like you to do is to get two pieces of string, each about five feet long. Don't continue reading until you've gotten them.

Got the strings? Good. Now, take one of them and put it down on the floor in the shape of a circle. Imagine that the circle is the size of your waist, and using *only* your imagination, adjust the size of the circle to the size you believe your actual waist to be.

Now take the second string and put it around your waist to measure the real circumference. When you've got it, lay *this* string down next to the first one.

What did you find? Surprised? I'll wager that the waist of your imagination is bigger than your actual one.

Was I right? And just how did I know that you would literally have an inflated sense of yourself? Although I'd love to possess mystical powers, the truth is that I could predict that the circle of your imagination would be bigger than the accurate one because virtually everyone in my program carries around the same mental distortions.

❧

The best way out is always through.

—ROBERT FROST

I asked you to do this exercise to make the point that in the most basic, physical way, we carry ideas around in our head of *who we are*. Left unchallenged, these ideas about ourselves, this script that we formed early on, will largely determine how we interact with the world. Our script will profoundly affect the way we present ourselves to others. The way we present everything out there to ourselves. And when our self-image, the core set of ideas about who we are, is distorted in a negative way, all bad things will *naturally* follow. Unwittingly, we play an active role in shaping our own miserable destinies.

An event in Mary's life puts flesh on all this abstract talk. As Mary described it, she was working her shift at the hospital when a supervising nurse came over and began to berate her publicly for "failing" to complete some paperwork on time. Never mind that there had been several emergencies that day or that Mary had had to double for another nurse who'd called in sick at the last minute. The supervisor was having none of it. She was infamous for her unfairness and verbal abuse, and no one yet had figured out a way to disarm her.

So Mary stood there in the hall, taking in the scolding, barely saying anything before returning to her patients. At the end of her shift, Mary slipped out of the hospital as quickly as she could. She did not stop to exchange customary good-byes with coworkers. She did not do this because Mary was already in her trance state and heading for the grocery. Once there, she bought pretzels. She bought cookies. She bought ice cream. And then she went to the home she knew would be empty because her husband always got home late on Tuesdays and she ate them all. Watching TV. Alone.

Sound familiar?

Let's go back now to the beginning of this morose piece of Mary's movie and see what we can learn from blowing up each frame. We begin with what we might call a *situation* or *event*. In this case, the event is Mary's boss berating her in public. Sometimes we can misinterpret another person's behavior, but let's assume that in this instance, there was no confusion. Mary's supervisor absolutely, unequivocally, berated her publicly. "And I just stood there and took it," said Mary, her tone still defeated. "I mean, I tried to say a few things in my defense, but she just ran over me like a bulldozer. That's the way she is."

Let's stop the action right here for a moment. Mary is standing in the hall. She is being blamed, loudly and in front of other people. And while this is going on and immediately after, Mary is very aware that

Thoughts are energy, and you can make your world or break your world by thinking.

—SUSAN TAYLOR

this scene is being acted out in public. She is having *thoughts* about what is going on.

I can't emphasize enough how important it is that we understand that the first thing Mary has are thoughts. These are the things we tell ourselves in our heads, and they often pass through so quickly that we're not even aware of them. What we are on much more familiar terms with are the *feelings* that follow. These are the emotions, what we experience on a "gut" level that can so quickly flood us.

But first come the thoughts. And what were Mary's?

Her first thought: "People are watching me."

Mary is not a journalist here, observing the event in a neutral way. She is a player, and she attaches great meaning to what is happening. She makes that clear by describing herself as "just standing there."

Her next thought: "I'm not standing up for myself."

When Mary thinks she has not stood up for herself, of course, she is telling herself that she's a coward. She is telling herself that a "better" person would or should have reacted differently.

Her final thought: "I didn't do my job."

Regardless of the "evidence," Mary thinks that perhaps her supervisor was right. "I mean, rationally I know I was doing a good job, but you know me well enough by now to know there's always a part of me that worries about whether I'm doing enough for others."

"To me," Brendan jumps in, barely able to contain himself, "the humiliation of being yelled at while others are watching and not standing up for yourself is the whole story. Believe me, I should know. Every day growing up with my father was like that."

"I didn't have an abusive father," Mary responds, "but there's no question about it, I felt that I hadn't stood up for myself."

Actually, Mary didn't *feel* she hadn't. She *thought* she hadn't. I make this distinction not to split verbal hairs but because understanding the *sequence* of what goes on is essential if we are to follow Mary's journey to unhappiness. Mary *thinks* she hasn't stood up for herself. She then has certain *feelings:* "Like I said, I felt humiliated. I don't know if it's the same or not, but I felt embarrassed. Ashamed."

Humiliation. Embarrassment. Shame. These are the *feelings* that follow

We have met the enemy and he is us.

—WALT KELLY (*POGO* CREATOR)

Mary's thoughts. Put yourself in Mary's shoes now and try to identify
what other feelings she might be experiencing:

_____

_____

_____

_____

Brendan: "If anxiety is a feeling, I'd be feeling that."

Mary: "I won't deny that I felt very anxious while it was happening."

Fern: "How about anger? When things like that happen to me, I feel blind rage afterward."

Mary: "I'm not like Fern in that way. If I was feeling angry, I'd probably be the last person to know it."

Some of the feelings my workshop participants cited were *hopeless, depressed, frustrated, guilty,* and *sad.*

Mary: "I'm sure I felt all of those things."

So we began with an event. How Mary interpreted the event, her thoughts, led to specific feelings. The next question is, What does Mary do with these feelings? How does she react to her feelings, not internally, but with acts, with specific *behaviors?*

I think there are three distinct pieces of behavior that come in the wake of Mary's feelings:

1. She leaves work as quickly as she can without saying good-bye to anyone, completely negating herself.
2. She goes to the grocery store and buys junk food, sending a further message of her worthlessness.
3. She goes home and eats in solitude, sealing her lonely fate.

These are the three things that Mary *does.* On one level, she understands her behavior. "I left work quickly to avoid other people because I felt humiliated. I bought junk food because that's what I usually do, although this was more intense. And what I'm learning, I suppose, is that when I go into that trance state of compulsive eating, I'm tranquilizing my feelings with food."

But there's more. When Mary is done eating, when the last cookie

The hues of the opal, the light of the diamond, are not to be seen if the eye is too near.

—RALPH WALDO EMERSON

has disappeared and she can't scrape one more sliver of ice cream from the bottom of the container, the tranquility takes an ugly turn. "I tell myself I'm a failure. That I'm out of control. What's wrong with me? Why can't I take charge of myself? I feel terrible. Disgusted with myself."

Mary ends up feeling the same after eating as she did after the run-in with her boss. Now let's widen the lens. If your thoughts about yourself and the feelings that follow after you've eaten compulsively are similar to what you thought and felt after being humiliated, how do they compare with the way you think and feel about yourself at other times?

What core set of beliefs about yourself, the ones you carry around buried deep inside you, are being played out as you relive the original pain through a cycle of bingeing that reliably ends in self-recrimination? You know, what's popularly referred to as your self-image. How does it compare with the world you lived in as a child?

For Mary, who didn't even feel entitled to criticize her upbringing, one core belief emerged as dominant: She was supposed to take care of everyone else. The messages people received about themselves were echoed over and over in my treatment groups:

> *I'm not important.*
> *Everyone else's needs come before mine.*
> *I'm not good enough.*
> *I'm not supposed to get angry.*
> *I'm bad.*

Mary agrees that all these thoughts resonate for her. Now just imagine the implications of this incredibly powerful system of core beliefs reinforced thousands of times as you eat to soothe yourself, then turn it against yourself. When you think of the way you feel after you've been humiliated or dismissed or after you've binged, is that very different from the way you thought and felt after someone in your family put you down? Or, as in Mary's case, she was always taking care of others, yet emotionally was alone.

We'll be returning to that childhood kitchen many times. For now, perhaps it's enough to note how amazing it is the way, as adults, we keep writing scripts that emanate from the core beliefs about ourselves

❧

I dance to the tune that is played.

—SPANISH PROVERB

we developed oh, so many years ago and then unconsciously, mysteriously recapitulate and validate those original beliefs. You can release us anywhere and, like homing pigeons, we'll find a way to get back to where we started.

Mary's *event* gives rise to *thoughts,* which in turn create *feelings* that result in specific *behaviors.* The consequence is that Mary feels really terrible about herself. The tragedy is that she doesn't even have the opportunity to assess the situation and react with any perspective before the vicious cycle kicks in. If Mary weren't so absolutely certain that she was worthless, she might have more optimistic thoughts. Mary cannot control how she "should" feel, but it's important that we understand that there is no other way she *could* feel, given the messages she's received and the way she's reinforced those negative messages thousands of times with food.

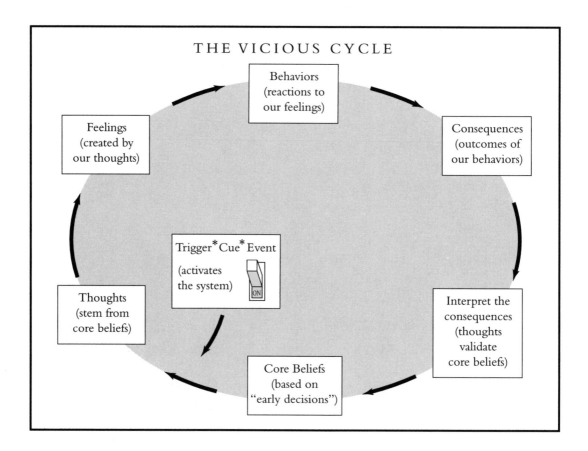

THE VICIOUS CYCLE

Behaviors
(reactions to
our feelings)

Consequences
(outcomes of
our behaviors)

Feelings
(created by
our thoughts)

Trigger * Cue * Event
(activates
the system)

Interpret the
consequences
(thoughts
validate
core beliefs)

Thoughts
(stem from
core beliefs)

Core Beliefs
(based on
"early decisions")

Let's put a different pair of lenses on our Mary now and see if the vicious cycle she follows has to be as invariable as the earth's orbit of the sun—whether there's anything she might be able to do for herself. The scene again is the hallway of the hospital. Mary is being yelled at by her supervisor. Coworkers are nearby. And Mary is thinking, "People are watching. I'm not standing up for myself. I didn't do what I was supposed to do."

When I asked my workshop participants to chip in, it was Fern who broke the ice: "The one thing I keep thinking is what a _____ (expletive deleted) idiot Mary's boss is."

Likewise, it's possible that the coworkers are thinking more about what a miserable person the boss is than about Mary not standing up for herself. Or about how they felt when the supervisor abused them, since she's apparently an equal-opportunity creep and nobody yet has figured out what to do about her.

It is clearly Mary's script that tells her she's a failure. If she were able to grant herself some thoughts that were more like strokes than put-downs, she might not feel as self-conscious. If she didn't think of herself so much as a failure, she would undoubtedly feel less helpless and depressed.

Fern: "It just struck me that if I couldn't stand up to my boss because she was the boss and no one could, and if I thought everyone else was thinking what a bitch she was, I might not even feel so angry. I'd certainly feel stronger and more successful."

Brendan: "Maybe not happy, but certainly less depressed."

But Mary has a hard time imagining even getting to that place, which brings us back to the change we were talking about last week and how scary it is even when it's change for the better. I asked Mary to visualize herself walking out of the hospital with better thoughts and feelings about herself.

Mary: "I wish I could say I would have gone home and had carrot juice and spinach, but I think I'd be lying to myself. I eat junk food compulsively. At other times, there doesn't necessarily have to be a trigger event."

This may be one of the biggest frustrations of all for compulsive eaters. The eating is pandemic. It's impossible, it seems, to identify "reasons" for binges if we find ourselves bingeing all the time.

As he thinketh in his heart, so is he.

—PROVERBS 23:7

However, Mary did say she ate more than usual that night. And that's a start.

I'd like you to pay very close attention to events that trigger more bingeing. If you have an especially bad or out-of-control eating experience, break it down in the following way: Describe the *event* that occurred, the *thoughts* or *interpretation* you gave to it, the *feelings* that followed, your subsequent *behavior,* and the *consequences* in terms of where that left you in relationship to yourself.

Before you begin, let me offer an example from Fern's chart just to give you a sense of how it goes:

Fern's Record of Thoughts

The Situation

The meanings of things lie not in the things themselves but in our attitude towards them.

—ANTOINE DE SAINT-EXUPÉRY

Describe the Event: A guy I was supposed to go out with on a second date left a message on my answering machine that something had come up at the office and he had to cancel.

The Thoughts: He didn't really like me. Someone he liked better had become available at the last minute. Men are all alike. I don't know why I even bother to try.

The Feelings: First and foremost, anger. Mostly at him. Then at my mother, who called to see how the date had gone. Maybe some depression.

The Behavior: Five jelly doughnuts. Then I punished myself by making myself sleep on the couch instead of in bed.

The Consequences: Fury at myself for still giving a damn about whether a guy takes me out or not, and of course for eating all those doughnuts.

Anger, at others and at herself, is Fern's old friend. So that's her cycle, her life script. Now it's your turn. Using the chart on the next page, take yourself through one cycle using the enclosed Record of Thoughts chart:

RECORD OF THOUGHTS

Situation	Automatic Thoughts	Feelings	Behavior	Consequences
Describe the event	Your interpretation of the event	In response to thoughts	Your reaction	Outcome as a result of actions

How did you make out? Did you get some sense of how you play the sad game of *negative reinforcement?* I hope so. Your homework is to take at least three other events that occur in the next week and fill in the steps that follow for each one.

Then (I think you know what's coming) I want you to go through the cycle by substituting some different, more generous thoughts, and see where *they* take you.

FOOD FOR THOUGHT

WEEK FIVE

Days One Through Six

Identify an event that occurred today and follow it through the cycle— event, thoughts, feelings, behavior, consequences—using the enclosed Vicious Cycle Worksheet.

Day Seven

Today, go back to the daily worksheets for Days One through Six. Using a different color pencil, substitute stroking thoughts for any put-down thoughts you listed in the past six days. Now follow the new thoughts through the cycle. Where do they take you?

_____

_____

Weekly Checklist

____ 1. Did you complete the string exercise?

____ 2. Did you fill in the Record of Thoughts chart?

____ 3. Did you keep a daily record of trigger events and their consequences using the Vicious Cycle Worksheet?

____ 4. Have you stayed aware of physical versus nonphysical hunger?

THE VICIOUS CYCLE WORKSHEET

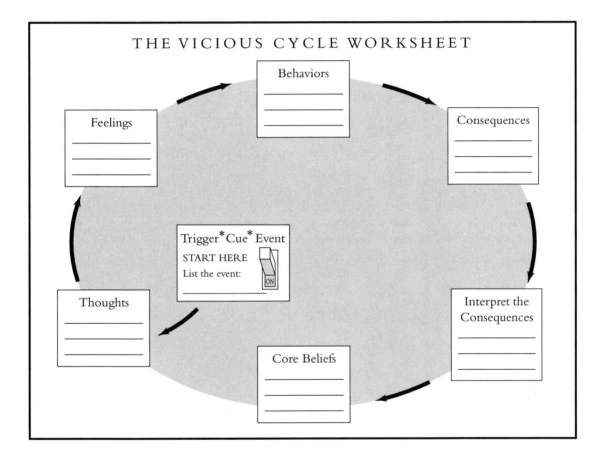

Behaviors
_____
_____
_____

Consequences
_____
_____
_____

Feelings
_____
_____
_____

Trigger*Cue*Event
START HERE
List the event:
_____

Interpret the Consequences
_____
_____
_____

Thoughts
_____
_____
_____

Core Beliefs
_____
_____
_____

THE VICIOUS CYCLE WORKSHEET

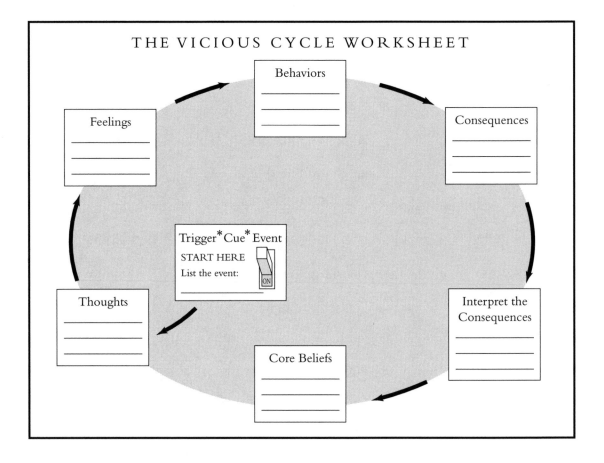

Behaviors
_____
_____
_____

Consequences
_____
_____
_____
_____

Feelings
_____
_____
_____

Trigger*Cue*Event
START HERE
List the event:
ON
_____

Interpret the
Consequences
_____
_____
_____
_____

Thoughts
_____
_____
_____
_____

Core Beliefs
_____
_____
_____

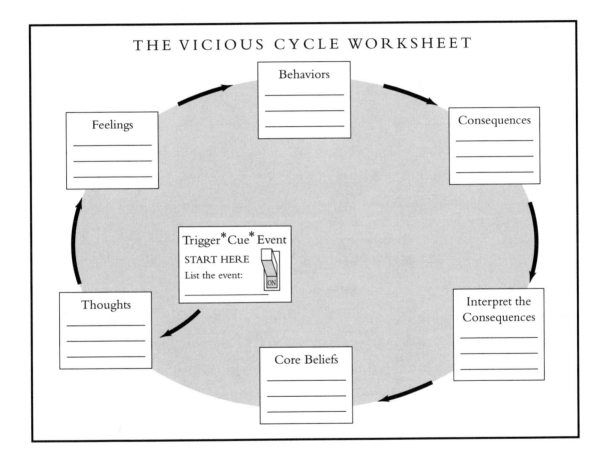

THE VICIOUS CYCLE WORKSHEET

Behaviors

Feelings

Consequences

Trigger*Cue* Event
START HERE
List the event:
ON

Thoughts

Interpret the Consequences

Core Beliefs

THE VICIOUS CYCLE WORKSHEET

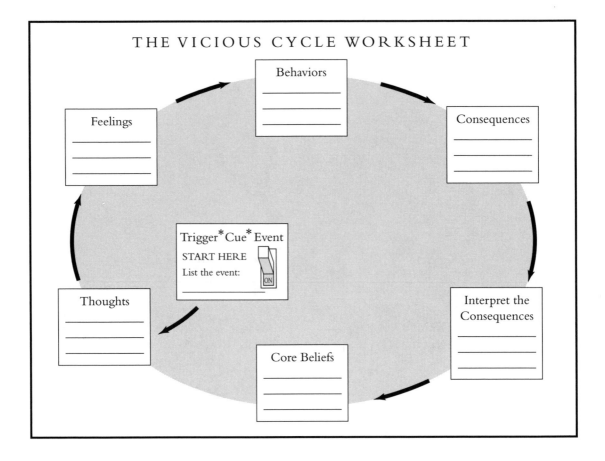

Behaviors
_____
_____
_____

Consequences
_____
_____
_____

Feelings
_____
_____
_____

Trigger*Cue* Event
START HERE
List the event:
_____ [ON]

Interpret the
Consequences
_____
_____
_____

Thoughts
_____
_____
_____

Core Beliefs
_____
_____
_____

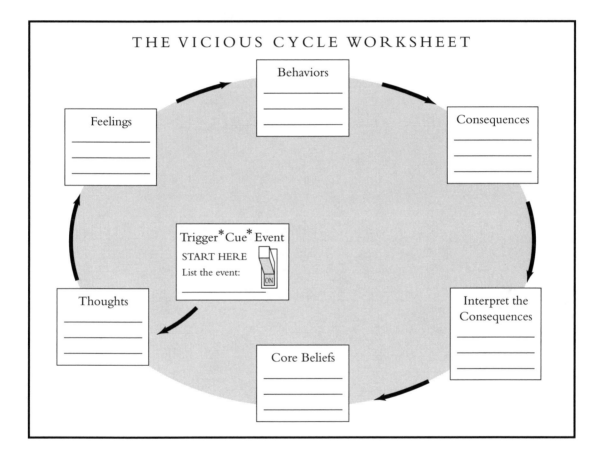

THE VICIOUS CYCLE WORKSHEET

Behaviors

Feelings

Consequences

Trigger*Cue* Event

START HERE

List the event:

ON

Thoughts

Interpret the
Consequences

Core Beliefs

THE VICIOUS CYCLE WORKSHEET

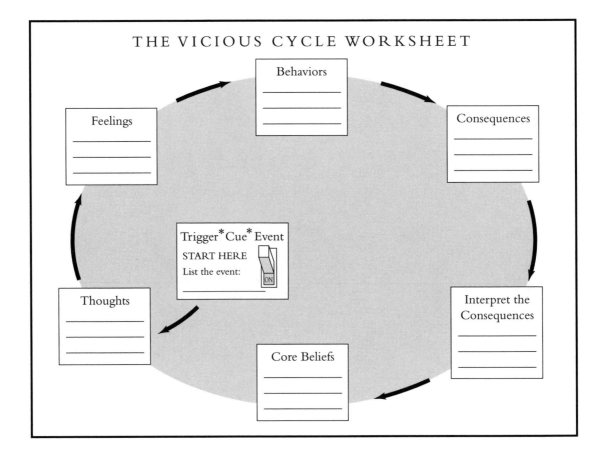

Behaviors
_____
_____
_____

Feelings
_____
_____
_____

Consequences
_____
_____
_____

Trigger *Cue* Event
START HERE
List the event:
_____ ON

Thoughts
_____
_____
_____

Core Beliefs
_____
_____
_____

Interpret the
Consequences
_____
_____
_____

Forbidden Fruit

❧

Grab your emotional taste buds. If you thought a potato chip was only a potato chip, this week's menu will give you more than food to digest.

Ready for a change of pace? I hope so, because this week we're going to be, as people who are always dieting put it, *bad*. That's right. We're going to eat the things we're *not supposed to*. We're going to open our mouths and see how our emotional tastebuds respond.

But first a word from our sponsor. I would like it so much if you would spend a few minutes now going back to what got us to this point. Specifically, take a U-turn to your Hunger Awareness Diary and Strokes and Put-Downs Worksheet of Week Two. Review what you recorded and sift through it again. Add anything new that might come to mind now. Then have a brief reunion with the genogram information you put together in Weeks Three and Four. Refresh your memory. Add new material that may have surfaced.

Finally, how about your Record of Thoughts? Did you take yourself through a cycle? Were you able to substitute some different thoughts and see where they took you? If not, how about doing it now? When Brendan (a week late, but who's counting?) did it, here's what his first and second versions looked like:

❧

A matter that becomes clear ceases to concern us.

—Friedrich Wilhelm Nietzsche

Brendan's Record of Thoughts

The Situation

My sister practically ignored me at a dinner party.

The Thoughts: She doesn't really love me. She's angry at me. I have a screwed-up family. Nobody's there for me.

The Feelings: Sad. Anxious. Lonely. Abandoned (even though you wouldn't have known it if you had seen me being the life of the party). Guilty (I must have done something wrong, even if I don't know what).

The Behavior: I never let the peanuts get out of my reach. I talked a lot (even for me!). I left without saying good-bye to my sister (I guess I must have also felt some anger).

The Consequences: I'm not sure, other than I felt lousy about myself and when I went to sleep I had a nightmare in which I had started drinking again.

Brendan's Record of More Generous Thoughts (written the following day)

Paralyze resistance with persistence.

—WOODY HAYES

The Situation

The same.

More Generous Thoughts: My sister didn't mean to ignore me. She kissed me when I first arrived. We had spoken by phone for over an hour two nights before and she wanted to circulate with new people, especially the guy she was talking with. I would have wanted to do the same with an attractive woman.

The Feelings: Much better. Optimistic. Strong. Connected.

The Behavior: This may sound like an infomercial, but I actually didn't overeat that night. At least not much. I called my sister and we talked and—surprise, surprise—of course she wasn't angry at me, but I'm glad I called so my imagination didn't get the better of me.

The Consequences: Needless to say, I felt better after hearing my sister's reassuring voice and after wading, not diving, into food last night.

I want to be very clear here to let you know that Brendan has not just experienced a Miracle Cure like those we see falsely advertised all the time. His emotional relationship with food will not reverse itself overnight. Nor should it! A major reason that quick-weight-loss diets are a disaster is that our bodies will eventually "rebel" against significant deprivation. Emotional change that is too fast will produce the same effect. Regardless of how "good" that change is, it will feel painfully uncomfortable if we take more of a bite than our system can comfortably digest.

Taking the initiative to entertain different thoughts *did* lead Brendan to different feelings. Those new feelings took him from reaching for carbohydrates to reaching for the phone, a reassuring talk with his sister, a night of normal eating, and satisfaction. What Brendan did was *begin*. And I hope you did too!

What I want to do this week is take what we've been talking about and show you how it translates into our direct experience with food. We're going to do this through a tasty exercise that I know you'll enjoy. What you'll need is the following:

1 grape
1 potato chip
1 chocolate kiss
1 glass of water

I realize that you may not have some of the items around, so I'll be happy to wait while you go out and buy them or find reasonable substitutes. After you've assembled everything, I'd like you to start by laying out each food item in front of you so they don't touch. Have a pencil ready to record what you're about to experience in the chart on the next page:

Things sweet to taste prove in digestion sour.

—WILLIAM SHAKESPEARE

EATING AWARENESS EXERCISE

Food Item	Automatic Thoughts Your interpretation of the food item	Feelings In response to thoughts	Behavior Your reaction	Consequences Outcome as a resut of actions

Start with the grape. Hold it in your hand. Don't put it into your mouth yet. Just keep looking at it. What are the thoughts that come into your head? Here are a few that occurred to Fern, Brendan, and Mary:

Fern: "It feels cool. I never really focused on the color of a grape before. This green reminds me of the color of a river I saw once in Central America."

Brendan: "One grape? What can I do with one grape? They make wine from grapes. I wish I could drink again."

Mary: "I wonder how sweet this will taste. You never know. Grapes can be sweet as sugar or very tart. I hope this one is sweet."

Get the idea? Okay, how about entering a few thoughts of your own in the Eating Awareness Exercise Worksheet?

What I'd like you to do next is to put the grape into your mouth without biting down on it yet. Just hold it there on your tongue with your mouth closed. As you're doing this, jot down your thoughts in the worksheet. What does the grape feel like against your tongue? Is it cool? Can you taste any sweetness? How does it feel against your teeth? Your upper and lower palates? Do you sense the salivary glands in the back of your throat starting to secrete? These are the things I want you to focus on.

Slowly, slowly now, bite into the grape. Whatever you do, don't swallow it. Keep the grape in your mouth as long as you can. Try to experience the subtle shifts of flavor as you gently chew it. Write down what you're *feeling* while you do this.

Finally, swallow the grape, but as you swallow it, see how far you can follow it down your throat. Actually, travel with it as it makes its way down and enters your esophagus. Write out your thoughts and feelings.

Okay, so what did we come up with as a result of this one-grape experience?

Fern: "I found it crunchy and too tart. Also, I had to swallow it before you said to swallow it because my salivary glands started to take over and make a big production of everything. I mean, I don't really even like grapes, and it just seemed like it was time for the grape to go down."

Brendan: "At first, the feeling was very smooth. Smooth and bland. Then when I began to salivate and bite, it changed to tangy, sour, slimy.

It's often the last key on the ring that opens the door.

—PROVERB

The skin is really tough. This may sound weird, but I enjoyed this grape less than any other I've eaten before."

Mary: "At first it tasted good, but then I felt I wanted more juice. And when I bit it and the juice came out onto my tongue and I didn't swallow, it started to taste bad. I think part of the problem was that we had to be aware of what we were experiencing all the time."

Exactly. This was the beginning of our Eating Awareness Exercise. The only question is whether the "problem," as Mary calls it, is her awareness of what she was eating, or is it that when we eat compulsively, we have absolutely *no* awareness of what we're shoving into our mouths? If you always ate grapes this way, how many do you think you would eat at a time?

Mary: "One. Maybe two."

Right. Research shows that when people become conscious of every mouthful of food—if they really pay attention to what's going on—they eat less. *Much* less.

Fern: "But this doesn't seem to me to be a natural way to eat. Nobody I know would sit with one grape in their mouth waiting for their salivary glands to do whatever. And how about those lionesses you like to talk about? I've seen the nature documentaries of them feeding, and *they* sure don't dwell on each tiny morsel of warthog, experiencing all the subtle changes in their taste buds."

They sure don't. They tear in to their food. But as you know from watching them, the lionesses eat to satisfy their hunger. Because food has no other meaning to them, when they're done, they're done. I'm sure you've never seen a lioness finish off her main course and almost immediately head out looking for a late-night snack. The only thing that will get a lioness hunting for food is physical hunger. And to a large extent, as we know, healthy human eaters operate the same way.

Back now to our exercise. Here's what Mary's worksheet looked like:

I'm a slow walker but I never walk back.

—ABRAHAM LINCOLN

FOOD ITEM	THOUGHTS	FEELINGS	BEHAVIOR	CONSEQUENCES
One grape	Healthy food Will it be sweet?	Safe	Eat the grape	Not that satisfied with food Didn't feel anxious I was a "good" girl

How about yours? If you're like most people (Brendan's being reminded of wine is a notable exception), the experience of eating the grape was a relatively benign one. Now let's move on. Pick up the potato chip, and hold it in your hand. Just keep holding it and looking at it. Then write down any thoughts you have.

When you've finished writing, I'd like you to take the potato chip, just as we did with the grape, and put it into your mouth and take a bite out of it. Don't chew the piece you've bitten off. Just hold it in there. As you're doing this, write down how it feels. What are you tasting? Do you feel your salivary glands secreting with the potato chip? How does it feel against your teeth? What's happening in your mouth as you hold that potato chip in there? What's going on in your mind? What are you thinking with that potato chip in your mouth?

Start to bite into it now. Start chewing it, but don't swallow. Keep it in your mouth as long as you can. As you do, note if there are any changes in the taste and in the texture the longer it's there. What happens to that potato chip?

When you do swallow it, see if you can follow the potato chip as it's traveling down your throat and your esophagus. See how far you can accompany it. Write down what's going on in your head.

Done? Good. So what have we got here? What kinds of thoughts did our "eating a potato chip" event elicit?

Mary: "I was thinking that this is a bad food. I was thinking that I can't just eat one of these, that I can't control myself with potato chips. I'm addicted to them."

Given Mary's thoughts, what feelings would you guess might follow? By the way, when Mary says she is "addicted" to potato chips, do you think that is the case? There is, after all, no governmental agency I

The secret of success is to start from scratch and keep on scratching.

—PROVERB

know that labels potato chips an addictive substance. Yet Mary is completely sincere when she uses that word. The truth, I would suggest, is that Mary's addiction is not to the potato chip but to the feelings that come along with it. The same old feelings. And given Mary's thoughts, it's not hard to predict the kind of feelings that follow: anxiety, fear, and helplessness.

Brendan: "I don't know what else Mary could possibly feel. I mean, when they created that damn commercial about how you can't only eat just one potato chip, they knew what they were talking about."

You bet they did. Potato chips are sometimes referred to as a "trigger food," or something that sets off a feeding frenzy. And when you give this incredible power to the potato chip, when your thoughts tell you that it's the potato chip, not you, that has the power, you may have created a lose/lose situation for yourself. If you eat one, you eat the bag and end up beating up on yourself in that old, familiar way. If you decide you can't handle one and stay away, what consequences might occur?

Mary: "For me, I think I'd be really proud of myself to have that kind of discipline. I'd feel strong."

Probably. But there might be some other, less desirable consequences, and we'll get to them shortly. For now, how does your worksheet look for the potato chip?

Here's what Fern's looked like:

FOOD ITEM	THOUGHTS	FEELINGS	BEHAVIOR	CONSEQUENCES
One potato chip	Greasy Bad food I want it I have no control	Nervous Afraid Excited Resentful	Ate one	Felt guilty Felt fat Wanted more

How about your chart? Similarities? Differences? Does it strike you as amazing how one little potato chip can touch off so much in us? How clear it is that it's not about potato chips. Sure, salt can stimulate the appetite of all eaters, but someone else might recognize this and get a hit of salt from a more containable food item. With Fern, as we might surmise by now, that bag of potato chips takes her back to

We conquer not in any brilliant fashion. We conquer by continuing.

—CHARLES GEORGE MATHESON

the kitchen of her childhood, to the food her mother controlled, to the secret late-night raids with her father, and, most important, to the familiar feelings she keeps re-creating as an adult.

Ready for something sweet? Okay, clear your palate with some water, take out the chocolate kiss, and, without unwrapping it, hold it in your hand. Looking at it, what comes to mind? My first thought is how brilliant Hershey's was to call it a kiss. What wonderful associations most of us have with that word. Can you imagine our response if they had called it a blob?

Mary: "The thought that comes to mind is how it looks like a present wrapped in foil. I think of Christmas and gifts. Something you would have in a bowl for special occasions. It's so festive."

So even before we begin, there's a lot of big-time thinking going on. With Mary, her first thoughts are all positive ones. Fern's mind, on the other hand, took her in the opposite direction.

Fern: "We didn't celebrate Christmas in my family, so I don't have those associations. Actually, my first thought was 'It's lucky they have those things wrapped or I would eat them even faster.' Like with the potato chips, there's a sense that this is bad for me but I want it and once I start, I'm either out of control or I give up control. I'm not sure which."

Let's continue. Unwrap the kiss now and put it into your mouth. Let it sit there on top of your tongue. Take a small bite if you'd like or just let it melt. What does it feel like right now? Are your salivary glands secreting? Is it sweet? How does it feel against your tongue? Do you feel it up against your teeth? Write down the physical sensations and the feelings you're having. When you're ready, swallow what has melted or been chewed. As with the potato chip, see how far you can follow the chocolate down your throat and esophagus.

Done? Then have some water and let's talk about what your intimate encounter with the kiss was like.

Mary: "I let it melt in my mouth. At first it was very creamy and sweet, but then it started to taste more salty or bitter, I'm not sure which. I'm really astounded at how powerful my salivary glands are. I had no idea."

Fern: "I'm not sure whether it was creamy or sweet or what, but

Stolen sweets are always sweeter, Stolen kisses much completer.

—LEIGH HUNT

this was a very powerful emotional experience for me. I closed my eyes and as the chocolate dissolved, I was filled with this intense emotion. I almost started to cry. The word that comes to mind is 'longing.' Deep, deep longing. The emotions that came with the chocolate were more personal, more vulnerable."

Brendan: "I know what Fern means. For me, the potato chip was like having sex. The chocolate was like making love."

I can tell from the laughter and nodding heads that everyone knows exactly what Brendan means. By the way, how does your worksheet read on the chocolate event?

Brendan's worksheet:

❧

Nothing awakes a reminiscence like an odor.

—Victor Hugo

Food Item	Thoughts	Feelings	Behavior	Consequences
A chocolate kiss	Can't wait to eat it. I love chocolate I shouldn't eat it What's the point of this exercise?	Excitement Fear Guilt Confusion	Ate it	Lived to talk about it!

And you? What did you record on your worksheet for your close encounter of the chocolate kind?

Before we wrap it up for this week, I'd like to go back briefly to two things that were said earlier. The first is Mary's observation about how proud she'd feel if she ate only one potato chip. I said perhaps Mary would feel proud. But especially with the potato chip and chocolate kiss, I had the distinct impression that the anticipation of eating *only one* also left everyone feeling something less pleasant—*deprived*. And if we feel deprived, and the deprivation comes not from physical hunger but from emotional hunger, then what are we likely to do?

Fern: "I can read your mind. Eat secretly. Eat lots. Use food as a substitute. All the things we've been talking about."

You said it, Fern. And you can believe that when we go into our trance state and set out to fill our voids, it's not going to work for long for us to be "good" and abstain as we do with diets. When we diet and lose weight, we may be proud of ourselves, but if we're feeling deprived, we're a walking time bomb. It's only a matter of how long it is before we start looking for the potato chips and chocolate.

Clearly, then, if we're going to get anywhere with our compulsive eating, we have to deal with the feeling of emotional deprivation. We're going to have to find some way to strip food of the powerful meaning we give it. We need to find some other ways to feed ourselves emotionally.

A tall order, I know, but when Brendan compared potato chips to having sex and chocolate to making love, he was being more than clever with words. In his way, he was letting us know how big a deal food is for him. For us.

That, of course, was the point of this week's eating exercise. A grape. A potato chip. A chocolate kiss. The way we usually eat them, a few quick pops in the mouth. But slow up the action and put them under the microscope and we see that no way is a potato chip just a potato chip. As for chocolate . . . well, don't get me started.

Your homework is to take what we did this week and see how it relates to the cycle we talked about last week. In other words, how an event that doesn't involve an angry boss but a piece of food we put in our mouths takes us through the *same* cycle that ends up confirming the very core beliefs with which we started out.

What is food to one is to others bitter poison.

—LUCRETIUS

FOOD FOR THOUGHT

WEEK SIX

Day One

Think for a few moments. List the feelings that the thoughts of the following foods create for you:

Food	Feelings
mashed potatoes	_____
ice cream	_____
chicken soup	_____

pizza   _____

chocolate   _____

popcorn   _____

candy   _____

soda   _____

_____ (add some of your own)

Day Two

Categorize each of the foods listed into the columns below:

Dangerous	Yield	Go
"red light"	*"yellow light"*	*"green light"*
(stop!)	(proceed with caution)	(go)

Day Three

Choose one of your "green light" foods, practice taking a taste, and record your reactions.

1. What thoughts are going through your head? _____
_____

2. What feelings do your thoughts create? _____
_____

3. What eating behaviors do you find yourself engaging in? _____
_____

4. What are the consequences of these behaviors? _____
_____

Day Four

Choose one of your "yellow light" foods, practice taking a small taste, and record your reactions.

1. What thoughts are going through your head? _____
_____

2. What feelings do your thoughts create? _____
_____

❧

Ideas move fast when their time comes.

—CAROLYN HEILBRUN

3. What eating behaviors do you find yourself engaging in? _____
_____

4. What are the consequences of these behaviors? _____
_____

Day Five

Choose one of your "red light" foods, practice taking the smallest taste, and record your reactions.

1. What thoughts are going through your head? _____
_____

2. What feelings do your thoughts create? _____
_____

3. What eating behaviors do you find yourself engaging in? _____
_____

4. What are the consequences of these behaviors? _____
_____

5. Where does this "red light" food take you? _____
_____

A single idea, if it fits right, saves us the labor of an infinity of experiences.

— JACQUES MARITAIN

Day Six

Food, as we have seen in the previous exercise, is a vehicle we use to bring us back home to our "familiar territory." The emotional terrain we know. Identify three situations you can think of where you felt good (stroked) emotionally and where and how you used food to "bring you back home" (put yourself down), to take you back to that old familiar place—creating a put-down day. _____
_____

Day Seven

Go back to your Strokes and Put-Downs Tally Sheet from the previous weeks. List how often you used food to put yourself down: _____
_____

Describe the situations:_____
_____

Weekly Checklist

❧

*You have learnt some-
thing. That always feels at
first as if you had lost
something.*

—George Bernard Shaw

____ 1. Did you complete the Eating Awareness exercise?

____ 2. Did you complete your Food for Thought writing exercises?

____ 3. Are you using the Vicious Cycle Worksheet from Week Five to analyze your trigger events? Following is a copy of the worksheet for you to use.

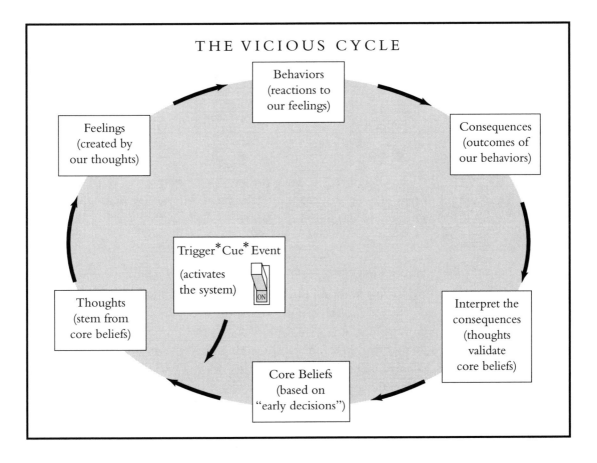

THE VICIOUS CYCLE

Behaviors
(reactions to
our feelings)

Consequences
(outcomes of
our behaviors)

Feelings
(created by
our thoughts)

Trigger*Cue* Event

(activates
the system) ON

Interpret the
consequences
(thoughts
validate
core beliefs)

Thoughts
(stem from
core beliefs)

Core Beliefs
(based on
"early decisions")

Casting Call

❧

Come backstage and meet the cast of the long-running show that keeps playing in your mind. See how well you know all their roles. Discover how many lines you've memorized.

❧

All the world's a stage, And all the men and women merely players: They have their exits and their entrances; And one man in his time plays many parts.

—WILLIAM SHAKESPEARE

You've probably heard the old riddle "How far into the forest can you go?" The answer is "Halfway. After that, you're coming out."

I congratulate you for having the strength to enter the gloomy forest of your compulsive eating for six weeks. You've reached the halfway point. From here on, you'll be emerging. If some of what we've been talking about, along with the exercises you've been doing, is starting to be helpful, great. If not, if you're struggling and not sure whether there's any way out of your food forest, I understand. I also urge you to stay with this. There's a way out of every forest.

Here's how Fern, Brendan, and Mary assessed themselves at this point:

Fern: "I'm angry. Angry and depressed. I had a bad week with food so it makes me wonder if I'm back at square one. I have to admit that at least I'm more conscious of what's going on. You mentioned a few weeks ago that often, when things are going well, we go back to our old comfortably miserable place . . . to what you call our script. Well, that's where I am this week."

Brendan: "Without going overboard, I'd say I'm feeling rather optimistic. I had several eating experiences this week that didn't feel compulsive, and believe it or not, I actually joined a gym [laughing]. Maybe next week I'll even go there and work out."

Mary: "I'm somewhere between Fern and Brendan. It's upsetting that there's no easy cure for this, yet I do feel that I'm learning so much. I carry these meetings away with me each week and I already have a whole notebook filled with things I hear at these meetings and with the exercises we do when we're home. That doesn't mean I have a firm grip on my eating, but something interesting happened last week on Thanksgiving that made me feel there might be some light at the end of the tunnel.

"Thanksgiving has been at my home for so many years that it's a tradition by now. Everyone relies on me to organize it all, which takes weeks of preparation. This year, what with my job, I had a brief fantasy about not doing it, but that would have disappointed everyone and, besides, part of me still wanted to.

"Without meaning to brag, I can say the dinner was a great success. I always get lots of compliments. When the last guest was gone and my husband was in the family room watching TV, I went into the kitchen to clean up and put away the leftovers. I had been so busy serving others that I hadn't eaten a thing. I found myself standing at the counter, nibbling away and wondering why I felt so empty inside. I knew from here that it wasn't just physical hunger.

"Remember how I once said I go on eating sprees at times when there is no negative event to trigger it, like the run-in with my supervisor I told you about a couple of weeks ago? Well, here was a perfect example. It had been a lovely day. I had gotten plenty of strokes. I had been surrounded by people who love me. Yet here I was, back in the kitchen, feeling alone, filling that emptiness with food.

"For a few seconds, my mind seemed to go blank. What came into my head next was that as nice as this day had been, I had done almost all the work. And I hadn't even asked for help. I think if I had asked people to bring different dishes, they would have been happy to. If I had asked for help serving or cleaning up, it would have been fine. In fact, some people asked if they could help and I said no. So there was old Mary, doing her same old providing thing, acting as though this was my preordained destiny in life.

The unexamined life is not worth living.

—PLATO

"What I did next shocked me. I put down the food, went into the family room, and cuddled up next to my husband. He acted surprised and asked if there was something else I wanted to watch. I almost said no, the football game was fine, but somehow I managed to suggest that maybe we could find a movie. We did. It was an old Bing Crosby movie, and we both really enjoyed it. During one of the commercials, I was about to ask him if he'd like me to get him some pie, when again I stopped myself and—get this—I asked him if he'd get *me* a piece. He must have been taken aback because that's so unlike me, but he came out of the kitchen with two pieces and he did this little bow and he was smiling.

"To top everything off, I only ate a couple of forkfuls. Then I put my plate down and cuddled up next to him again and we watched the rest of the movie. Later, he asked me if I wanted to go upstairs with him, if you know what I mean, and this was one night I didn't go to bed physically or psychologically hungry."

So there you have it. Three different voices. All important. And all ones we will get back to later this week. Now, how about you? What thoughts and feelings do you have about *your* progress to date? Spend a little time now thinking about how you're doing.

You'll recall that in Week Five (The Vicious Cycle), we talked about how our thoughts influence our feelings, which in turn determine our behavior, and how the consequence of all this is to complete the loop and bring us back home to reconfirm the core belief system we have about ourselves. Last week (Forbidden Fruit), we applied the same approach to specific food items: the grape, the potato chip, and the chocolate kiss.

What I want to do this week is help you get inside that loop to see what makes it go 'round and 'round. I want to bring you deep into your food forest. I want you to meet the *people* who keep giving you the directions that have you going around in circles. And I want to offer you a compass that you can use to point the way to sunlight.

I have no desire to turn this into a lecture in introductory psych, so I'll just briefly mention three expressions Freud coined, which I'm sure you've heard many times. They are, I think, a good way to open the curtain to your backstage cast.

The first of these words is "id." Simply (or oversimply) put, that's the infant or child we carry within us, the part that wants what we

It is hard to fight an enemy who has outposts in your own mind.

—Sally Kempton

want when we want it. Food. Sex. Things. We want our needs met, we want them met *now,* and we could care less about other people or *their* needs.

Sound bad? Selfish? Freud would say absolutely not. It's what we're born with, so how can it be selfish? If it's "bad," then do we call the lioness bad for killing the baby zebra? That cute little thing who was just born? Whose helpless mother is standing nearby?

Yet we do make these judgments all the time. We convene grand juries in our mind to determine whether to indict ourselves, and for what. We do this because of what Freud called the "Superego." An interesting word. If the id is all our uncensored primal ooze, the superego (it is derived from the Latin *super,* meaning "above," and *ego,* meaning "self") is what tells us right from wrong. It's our parent, our society, our religion, all rolled into one. Because Pinocchio was made of wood, he needed a Jiminy Cricket to help him make those distinctions. *We* carry Jiminy with us at all times. We let the lioness off the hook because she has no conscience and therefore can't make choices or act differently. But us? That's another story.

Finally, there is the "Ego." The ego is our consciousness. Standing between our id telling us what we want and our superego telling us what we can't have or shouldn't do or be, the ego is kind of a referee or arbiter. It is always positioned between the warring parties, working overtime to find a negotiated agreement. The ego doesn't take sides. It's the rational voice, which in its adult state is clear-headed, analytical. Like Sergeant Joe Friday in the old TV series "Dragnet," its motto is "Just the facts, ma'am."

End of refresher course. Now let's go backstage. The noted psychiatrist and author of the classic *Games People Play* Dr. Eric Berne suggests there are five characters in our play. The first two are parental. They are: the Problematic Parent and the Loving Parent.

In their extreme forms, these characters are polar opposites. The first lets us know how bad, inadequate, stupid, irrelevant, and unwanted we are. It is a voice that constantly puts us down or lets us know that we can get strokes only if we are a certain kind of child—invisible, obedient, helping, a good student . . . whatever.

Every one of us has a Problematic Parent in our cast. Those early-childhood experiences we've talked about determine how significant a role this parent has. Rather than talk abstractly about this character, let's bring it to life and give it some actual features. In the space below, draw

There is a period of life when we swallow a knowledge of ourselves and it becomes either good or sour inside.

—PEARL BAILEY

a picture that represents your Problematic Parent. Don't worry about being a Picasso. Just let it come out. To help get you started, let me show you the Problematic Parent Fern created.

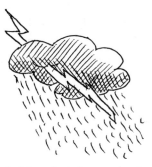

Got the idea? Good. Now let's have a look at yours.

MY PROBLEMATIC PARENT

Done? What did you come up with? Does your Problematic Parent have a gender? Remind you of anyone specifically? Any immediate associations you make when you look at what you have drawn?

Now that we have a glimpse of our Problematic Parent, let's give it some sample dialogue. These are the typical words or expressions that will follow it through the play. When I asked Brendan, Mary, and Fern for a characteristic line that might come out of the mouth of their Problematic Parent, here's what they came up with:

FERN'S PROBLEMATIC PARENT

"Can't you do anything right?"

BRENDAN'S PROBLEMATIC PARENT

"I'll show you who's the boss."

MARY'S PROBLEMATIC PARENT

"What's wrong with you!?"

If you'd like, you can spend a minute or two now thinking about your Problematic Parent's voice, but you'll be focusing on it and the other characters in your play more intensely in the daily exercises at the end of this chapter.

For now, let's move on to our second major character, the Loving Parent. If our Problematic Parent is the harshest possible superego, our Loving Parent, in its distilled form, is the audience who throws us bouquets of roses after each performance. It is the sound of an auditorium erupting in applause.

In the space below, create a picture of your Loving Parent. Again, don't focus on doing a "good" drawing, whatever that might be. Just relax and see what your pen or pencil brings forth.

In the carriages of the past, you can't go anywhere.

—MAXIM GORKY

MY LOVING PARENT

If you're finished with yours, take a look at what Brendan drew:

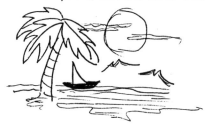

Now that you've gotten the picture, here's a piece of dialogue from Brendan's Loving Parent:

BRENDAN'S LOVING PARENT

"Don't pay him any mind. He doesn't know what he is doing. I'll give you the peace and comfort you need."

Enter the children. Just as there are two parental extremes (with many gradations in between), there are two archetypal inner children in our drama. The first of these is the Hungry Child.

An offspring of the Problematic Parent (remember, for our purposes, "problematic" does not have to mean overtly critical or physically abusive; it can include everything from withholding praise to significant physical and/or emotional absenteeism), the Hungry Child is a kind of orphan. And always, the Hungry Child operates out of fear. Fear of what? Of all forms of *negative parental judgments.*

You may remember in Week Two, Mary mentioned that when infants are almost completely deprived of Loving Parent input, they experience something called "failure to thrive" and literally die. We're talking here, of course, about something less extreme. Yet the emotional deprivation with which our Hungry Child emerges from childhood is hardly trivial. To survive at all, the Hungry Child has to adapt to a hostile or unwelcoming environment. The myriad ways she does so are truly amazing. The Hungry Child reminds me of trees that have somehow managed to grow in inhospitable terrain, over boulders, on cliffs, in the middle of rivers. Yet there they are, roots growing over the boulder, trunks leaning out over the cliff, branches stretching out over the river. Extraordinary!

And so it is with our Hungry Child. In the space below, introduce yourself to your Hungry Child by drawing a self-portrait.

Take care of the sense and the sounds will take care of themselves.

—LEWIS CARROLL

MY HUNGRY CHILD

Would you like to meet Mary's Hungry Child now? I hope so, because here she is:

Keep in mind as you think about the Hungry Child you've just drawn that all Hungry Children are not alike. They can take the form of a rebel or a goody-goody. Villain or victim. What they all share in common is a fear of the Problematic Parent. That fear is best illustrated by the lines of dialogue Mary wrote for her Hungry Child:

Experience is not what happens to you, it is what you do with what happens to you.

—ALDOUS HUXLEY

MARY'S HUNGRY CHILD

"I'm sorry. I didn't mean to make a mistake. I promise I'll do better the next time. Please forgive me."

The other child in our play, the opposite of the Hungry Child, is what I call the Nourished Child. This is the child who has been fed a strong diet of strokes. It is the child whose uninhibited id, filled with "I wants," has received plenty of encouragement. If the Hungry Child experiences the environment as unloving, the Nourished Child sees the world as her proverbial oyster. She is fearless, creative, spontaneous, curious. Again, this is an ideal. No child has all her needs met.

Draw your Nourished Child here.

MY NOURISHED CHILD

How does your Nourished Child compare with Fern's?

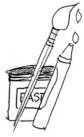

❧

Distance has the same effect on the mind as on the eye.

—SAMUEL JOHNSON

Just a reminder that you can begin to think about dialogue for each of your characters now, but you'll be doing the actual writing as Food for Thought exercises.

We're almost there. We have four of our featured players: the Problematic Parent, the Loving Parent, the Hungry Child, and the Nourished Child. Finally we come to the would-be star of our show. If this were the Academy Awards, the first four would be nominated under the category of Best Supporting Actor or Actress. This character wants to be the Best Actor or Actress in the Best Picture. It is the Adult.

It's no coincidence, I think, that the four other characters walk around carrying descriptive adjectives—"problematic," "loving," "hungry," and "nourished," while the Adult stands alone. That's because this character is the "just the facts, ma'am" part of our ego to which I referred earlier. No adjectives. No judgments. It's analytical. It's looking for optimal solutions. When we wrote our scripts very early in our lives, the adult ego state was not, could not, be present because it is not fully developed before the age of twelve. When we delete this character from our lives today, we emotionally return back to that time of parent-child interactions.

Based on the little I've given you to work with so far, draw a picture of the Adult that might be waiting in the wings of your stage.

MY ADULT

Brendan's Adult came out looking like this:

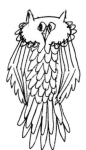

Earlier, I talked about how the Adult (*aka* the ego) looks not to judge but to observe and resolve. The entrance cue for the Adult comes when the Hungry Child and the Problematic Parent are onstage. That's the point, as we discussed in previous weeks, where *thoughts* follow an *event*.

For Mary, that was her reaction to being berated by her boss. For Brendan, you may recall, it was his sister not spending much time with him at a party. Fern's event was hearing a message on her answering machine that some guy was canceling a date. In every one of those events, the thoughts that followed were self-critical, the feelings negative, the behavior related to compulsive eating.

Fern, Brendan, and Mary all said that coming up with dialogue for their Adult was harder than for any of the other four characters. No wonder. If we had ready access to Adult dialogue, we wouldn't be compulsive eaters. The reason? Simple. If the Adult in you were, as the astrologists say, in ascension, it would intervene on your behalf in your problematic relationship with food.

Difficult as it was, Fern, Brendan, and Mary did come up with lines that related to their specific events. Here's Fern's Adult talking after the canceled date:

How many cares one loses when one decides not to be something but to be someone.

—Coco Chanel

FERN'S ADULT

"Why should I assume he has another date with someone he likes better? He said something had come up at the office. I have no prior evidence that he lies."

And Brendan's Adult sizing up his sister not talking to him much at a party:

BRENDAN'S ADULT

"My sister and I had talked for an hour on the phone the night before. She kissed me at the party when I arrived. She had told me in advance there was going to be a fellow there she was interested in. Why would I think she was angry at me?"

Finally, Mary's Adult taking charge as her boss berated her:

MARY'S ADULT

"Why should I feel bad? She does this to everyone. Nobody likes her. I may not be perfect, but I do my job as well as anyone. Is there any reason to think my coworkers don't know that?"

The way the Adult would, and will, surface on our behalf is the essence of what we'll be discovering in coming weeks. Before closing the curtain on this week, I'd like to mention that the five characters you carry around with you all the time have more than physical characteristics and lines to speak. Like all serious actors and actresses, they have a tone to their voice. They can also express themselves nonverbally. And they carry with them an attitude or mood state.

Below, I've put together a chart you can peruse when you get a chance. It lists each of the characters, or ego states, giving them the following abbreviations: Problematic Parent (PP), Loving Parent (LP), Adult (A), Nourished Child (NC), Hungry Child (HC). It also gives you a sampling of attributes that go with each. Study the chart and place yourself within it. Check off the qualities that describe your experience.

SOME IDENTIFIABLE CHARACTERISTICS OF EACH EGO STATE

	CP	NP	A	NC	AC
VERBAL EXPRESSION	bad should ought must always ridiculous	good kind I love you tender Good job You can do it	correct how? what? why? practical quantity logical	wow fun want ouch hi yea	I can't I wish try no I hope please I'm sorry I'm scared
TONE OF VOICE	critical condescending disgusted demeaning	loving comforting concerned encouraging	even concise balanced rational	free loud energetic	whiny defiant placating quiet shy
BEHAVIORS or NONVERBAL EXPRESSION	points finger frowns angry grimace ignoring punitive	open arms accepting smiling hug kiss listening	thoughtful alert open analytical problem-solving observing	uninhibited loose spontaneous adventurous inquisitive creative risk-taking	pouting rebellious acting out secretive withdrawn manipulative hiding compliant
ATTITUDE or MOOD STATE	judgmental moralistic authoritarian	understanding caring giving nurturing warm	erect matter-of-fact evaluation of facts	curious fun-loving changeable fearless happy content	demanding depressed ashamed fearful needy angry sad anxious

Adapted from: Woollams, S., Brown, M., Huige, K., Transactional Analysis in Brief, 1976.

Next week we'll get the five characters you've started to flesh out onto the stage and interacting. For now, a final word about this week. When Brendan, Mary, and Fern assessed themselves earlier, you heard Fern express anger and frustration because she had had a "bad" week around food. If you feel the same way at times, see if you can summon up the Adult in you to observe. The Adult is like a muscle in our body. It may be relatively unused, but it's there!

From here on, we're going to begin to exercise this muscle. We're going to make it stronger, more defined. With regard to your own eating, I think *your* Adult will lead you to a rational analysis of the facts and to the conclusion that over an extended period of time, the following will occur: There will be a decrease in the *duration* of your binges. There will be a decrease in the *intensity*. And there will be a decrease in the *frequency*. You'll see!

Identity is what you say you are according to what they say you can be.

—JILL JOHNSTON

FOOD FOR THOUGHT

WEEK SEVEN

Day One

Take a look at the drawing of your Problematic Parent. Describe this character: _____

_____

Day Two

Take a look at the drawing of your Loving Parent. Describe this character: _____

_____

Day Three

Take a look at the drawing of your Adult. Describe this character: _____

_____

Day Four

Take a look at the drawing of your Nourished Child. Describe this character: _____

_____

Day Five

Take a look at the drawing of your Hungry Child: Describe this character: _____

_____

Day Six

Go back to the pictures you drew for each of your characters. Write out examples of typical dialogue emerging from your:

Problematic Parent:_____

_____

Loving Parent: _____

_____

Adult: _____

_____

Nourished Child: _____

_____

Hungry Child: _____

_____

It is thus with most of us; we are what other people say we are. We know ourselves chiefly by hearsay.

—ERIC HOFFER

Day Seven

Look at the Problematic Parent dialogue that you generated in Day Six. Using your Adult voice, go back and challenge the Problematic Parent messages.

List Problematic Parent Messages: **List Adult Responses:**

_____   _____

_____   _____

_____   _____

Weekly Checklist

~

I'm not afraid of storms,
for I'm learning how to
sail my ship.

—LOUISA MAY ALCOTT

____ 1. Did you complete your drawing exercises?

____ 2. Did you complete your Food for Thought writing exercises?

____ 3. Are you using the Vicious Cycle Worksheet from Week Five to analyze your trigger events? Use the accompanying worksheet.

THE VICIOUS CYCLE WORKSHEET

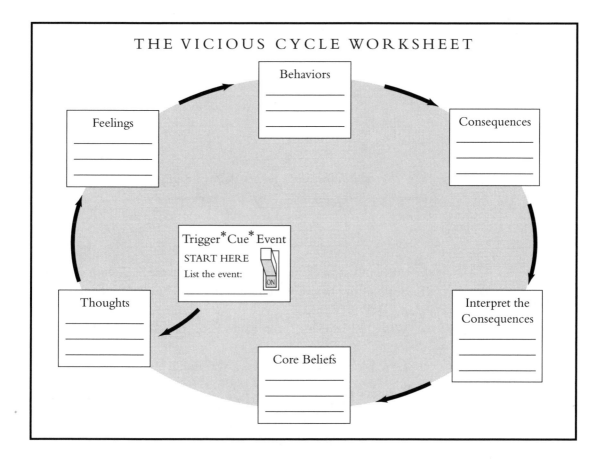

Behaviors
_____
_____
_____

Consequences
_____
_____
_____

Feelings
_____
_____
_____

Trigger*Cue* Event
START HERE
List the event:
_____
ON

Interpret the
Consequences
_____
_____
_____

Thoughts
_____
_____
_____

Core Beliefs
_____
_____
_____

Mirror, Mirror, on the Wall

❧

Now that you have put together your cast, it's time to bring in what they call a "play doctor." The first assignment? Create a new leading role.

❧

Our greatest foes, and whom we must chiefly combat, are within.

—MIGUEL DE CERVANTES

We left Fern last week in a bad state, but she came back with the words: "Reports of my failure were premature [laughing]. Oh thank you, my Adult."

What had happened to reassure Fern that all was not lost? Let her tell you:

Fern: "A couple of days ago, I was holiday shopping. While I was standing in line, I saw a pair of leggings I thought I could use. I asked the clerk to get me a pair. She asked if they were for me. When I said yes, she asked what size I was. I said I wasn't sure, a sixteen or an eighteen. Now, are you ready for this? The clerk rolled her eyes when I told her and said, shaking her head, 'Are you sure these are appropriate for someone your size?' "

When the group had stopped groaning in disbelief, Fern continued:

"Yeah, I know. But in the past I would have been so humiliated that I would have left all the things I had picked out right there and stormed out. This time, I somehow managed to catch myself. I actually took a deep breath and turned away for a second and pictured myself back here talking about the characters in our play. And lo and behold, out came my Adult and what it said to me was, 'It's her, not me.' The next thing you know, I picked up my packages, looked her right in the eye, and said, 'You just lost a sale . . . bitch.' Then I walked to the next counter and bought all my things."

Fern acknowledged the group's applause with a bow, and continued:

"Marilyn, I felt great! I said to myself, 'I did it! It works!' Normally, I would have gone home and eaten and cried myself to sleep. This time when I got home, I wrote a letter to the sales manager and mailed it in the morning on my way to work. I just hope I can hold on to this."

Brendan: "If you can, maybe you can bottle it for the rest of us. Actually, in its own way, what I did when I called my sister after the party was a little like your story. It's grabbing the bull by the horns. You simply didn't let that clerk get the best of you, Fern."

Mary: "I think what I did with my husband on Thanksgiving was similar, too, even though it involved asking for something and not expressing anger. But either way, it sure is nice to feel you can have some effect on what's around you."

It sure is.

The five characters who exist on all our stages, you'll recall, are the Problematic Parent, the Loving Parent, the Nourished Child, the Hungry Child, and The Adult. I don't think it will surprise you when I say that these characters don't need *others* to strut their stuff. They are constantly performing inside our own heads. And, as you can see, they also determine how we relate to *ourselves.*

The key to your sense of well-being, of course, is which characters you allow to take the leading roles. Do you have any control over who takes charge? You need to become aware of the dynamics, the situations where you cede control to a Problematic Parent or Hungry Child and when you stay with your Adult self.

In the diagram below, you'll find what is called an *egogram,* originally developed by psychotherapist Jack Dusay as a visual representation of how an individual appears to others. The five characters, beginning with the Problematic Parent, run across the bottom.

A bar graph is created for each character based on the relative importance or prominence each one represents in a given person's script at any time. This is a kind of collective graph that illustrates the typical

All you have to do is close your eyes and wait for the symbols.

—TENNESSEE WILLIAMS

or average response from the people in my workshops. Look at the graph carefully and pencil in how your graph might compare to the one below.

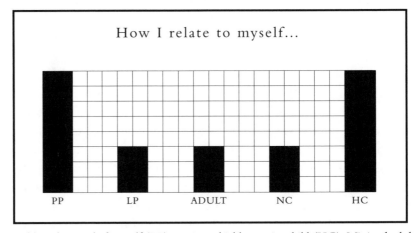

How I relate to myself...

PP   LP   ADULT   NC   HC

Highly judgmental of oneself (PP) creating a highly reactive child (HC). Minimal adult ego state present. You are playing out your "script" with yourself.

It is much easier to be critical than to be correct.

—BENJAMIN DISRAELI

As you can see, for the typical person, the cast members who perform most frequently in the play of how he or she relates to oneself are the Problematic Parent and Hungry Child. This pairing, needless to say, is not coincidental. You may have heard a song that begins, "It takes a worried man to sing a worried song." Well, just as surely, it takes a Problematic Parent to make a Hungry Child. These two characters act in consort with each other. It's what's known as a codependent relationship, in which one can't exist without the other. Soon you'll see how.

For now, let's get back to our graphs. This time I'd like you to look at the bars that depict the relative weight of each of the characters when it comes to how one relates to *others*.

With the people I work with in my groups, I actually found that the graphs take on one of two different looks. Here's the first:

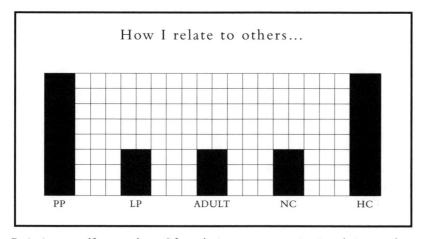

Projecting oneself onto others. Often playing out your script in relation to them. Minimal adult ego state present.

This one, as you can see, is identical to the How I Relate to Myself graph. In each instance, the Problematic Parent is dominant, either in our mind or in what we *project* onto others. In each case, the Hungry Child is equally present, highly reactive, judging itself negatively or critical of others. Just as important, the three characters who might bring some good energy onto the scene—the Loving Parent, the Nourished Child, and the Adult—are keeping a very low profile.

There is a second How I Relate to Others graph that I also see often, and it looks like this:

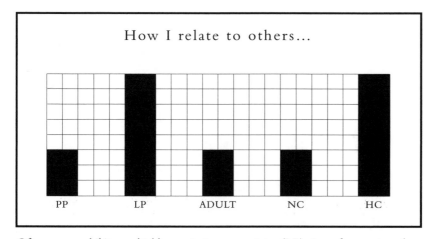

Often one exhibits a highly nurturing ego state (LP) in reference to others. Unconsciously seeking to be nurtured (HC) in return. Minimal adult ego state present.

∾

They who are to be judges must also be performers.

—ARISTOTLE

Notice the big difference? That's right. In this one, the Problematic Parent diminishes and the Loving Parent emerges. Want to guess how that might be a problem?

The problem is to be found in the bar at the far right of this graph. The Hungry Child is just as present as ever. This is the kind of emotional readout we would get from someone who is highly nurturing of others and unconsciously seeks to be nourished in return. On this stage also, there is very little Adult present.

Which of the two How I Relate to Others graphs most closely illustrates how you relate to others in your life? To your parents? Siblings? Colleagues? Boss? Friends?

From what you know of Fern, which one would you guess hers looks like? The first or the second? And Mary's? Similar or different?

If you chose the first graph for Fern and the second for Mary, you already know these women better than they knew themselves when they started the program. Fern certainly is critical of others *and* herself. Mary knows how to take care of others the way a great French chef knows how to make a sauce béarnaise. The problem with these graphs? Both Mary and Fern are going through life with emotional indigestion, the result of the dominant roles the Problematic Parent and Hungry Child play in our heads.

The exchange of dialogue between these two characters invariably contains all kinds of distortions of reality. For example, take a look at the following:

PROBLEMATIC PARENT

"I don't know why you even bother to sign up for a class. You won't follow through."

HUNGRY CHILD

"I guess you're right. What's the use? I can't do anything right."

When the Hungry Child says, "I can't do anything right," she has fallen into one of the most common "thought traps." Below are some of the major thought traps that snare people. Take a look at each one and see if it applies to *your* Problematic Parent and Hungry Child. Better still, try to recall a specific instance in which you play into your negative script.

COMMON THOUGHT TRAPS

1. Globalizing: You take a single negative event and turn it into a uiversal pattern of failure that characterizes your life.

Fern: "I guess I do this when I tell myself after a date doesn't work out that all men suck or that I'm 'destined' not to find a good one. I don't limit myself to that particular date or tell myself that this doesn't have to be my fate."

2. Either/Or Thinking: In the alphabet of your thinking, there is an A and a Z and nothing in between. If you do something that is less than perfect, you see yourself as a complete failure.

Mary: "I think this is a way I approach Thanksgiving. I have to do a million things, from shopping to cleaning up. It's hard for me even to imagine not doing everything. It's like in my head I either do it all or I'm somehow a failure."

3. Don't Confuse Me with the Facts: You come to negative conclusions about the meaning of events in your life even if there is no evidence to support your interpretations.

Brendan: "When I got into that thing about my sister not loving me because she didn't speak to me much at the party. Looking back at it, there really wasn't any evidence that she didn't love me but at the time, that was the immediate conclusion I drew."

4. I Plead Guilty: You are quick to blame yourself as the cause of some negative external event for which you are not, or not primarily, responsible.

Brendan: "I plead guilty. Over the weekend I got into a small fender bender at a traffic light. I automatically assumed it was my fault, and got

A lot of what acting is, is paying attention.

—ROBERT REDFORD

out of the car prepared to apologize. Imagine my shock when the other guy's first words were, 'Man, I'm sorry. I was trying to put in a CD and I lost my concentration for a second.' And I was ready to take full responsibility! The more I think about this, the more I think it's ridiculous to the point of being almost funny."

5. Accentuate the Negative: You blow up the significance of your mistakes so that they become as disastrous as the sinking of the *Titanic.*

Fern: "I can make a small mistake in writing up a contract and tell myself I'm too incompetent to be a lawyer, even though the contract is basically fine and people seem to respect my work. I am definitely my own worst critic."

6. Eliminate the Positive: You consistently find ways to trivialize your accomplishments while at the same time exaggerating the significance of anything anyone else achieves.

Fern: "I assume this is just the opposite side of the Accentuate the Negative coin. I do this all the time, too. I did it less than an hour ago when I heard someone say she had lost four pounds last week. As it happens, I lost two pounds, but instead of feeling good, my first thought was how well she was doing and how 'small' my accomplishment was."

7. But I Feel That Way: You live your life on the assumption that the negative feelings you have about yourself are as concrete and factual as your age, height, and eye color.

Mary: "I'm sure we all 'feel that way' or we wouldn't be here. When I feel (I guess you would say the right word is *think)* that my only role or value in life is as a provider or caretaker, I don't think that this is just an idea I have. I act like it's the gospel truth."

8. Wearing Magnifying Glasses: Like a teenager with one pimple, you take a single negative detail and blow it up so that it becomes the dominant feature in the way you view yourself.

Brendan: "I was sitting on a bus and I took up so much room on

Man's loneliness is but his fear of life.

—EUGENE O'NEILL

the seat that someone would have to have been a real skinny
Minnie to squeeze in next to me. No one did, so I quickly stood up,
and for the rest of the ride, I told myself that this was a metaphor for
my whole life, that in every way I take up too much space on this
planet."

9. Shoulda, Coulda, Woulda: You fill your thoughts with so many
"shoulds" and "shouldn'ts," not to mention "musts" and "oughts," that
the inevitable consequence is guilt when directed toward yourself,
anger when projected onto others.

Fern: "My whole life is filled with these, but the one that's probably
the most pervasive is this: I should have been a boy."

10. False Advertising: You are quick to label—or mislabel—yourself.
Instead of describing your behavior, you attach highly emotional, negative words to it. Billing yourself as A Failure is one of your favorite
headlines.

Mary: "I did that just this morning. I was in the supermarket, picking out oranges that were piled high in one of those bins. When I
reached for one, it started an avalanche. Maybe twenty came rolling
out onto the floor. I was mortified. And my first thought was, 'I
can't do anything right!' That's the way I labeled myself."

So? How many thought traps (Problematic Parent/Hungry Child)
did you fit "comfortably" into? Which ones were your "favorites"? Jot
them down now, make mental notes, or come back to these pages later
to see how they emerge as we move from scene to scene this week and
in weeks to come.

This might be a good time to take a short break, because there's an
exercise we're going to do now and you'll need a pen or pencil and
some writing paper.

Refreshed? Good. Here's what I want you to do. After you've read
this paragraph, close your eyes and *imagine* yourself standing naked in
front of a full-length, three-way mirror. Visualize yourself looking at all
parts of your body. Fantasize slowly turning around. As you do so, examine yourself closely. Pay particular attention to specific features with
which you are unhappy. As you continue to imagine yourself turning,

Listen to the voices.

—WILLIAM FAULKNER

begin to focus not only on what you see, but on the thoughts surfacing in your mind. Stop turning when you have selected the body part that displeases you most. Concentrate on the thoughts you are having as you zero in on that part. When you're done, open your eyes.

All right, now I'd like you to take the pencil or pen and, in the space provided below, write a letter to the body part you chose. That's right. A letter to that less-than-loved body part. Sound silly? Give it a try anyway. Write down all the thoughts you were having when your eyes were closed. Not sure how to begin? May I suggest:

Dear _____,

_____

_____

_____

_____

_____

_____

_____

_____

_____

_____

_____

_____

_____

_____

_____

_____

_____

_____

_____

_____

Finished? Okay, now take your pencil and place it in your nondominant hand (the one you *don't* write with). Give the body part you just wrote to a voice and, using your nondominant hand, write a letter from the body part you admonished back to yourself.

Where observation is concerned, chance favors only the prepared mind.

—LOUIS PASTEUR

_____

_____

_____

_____

_____

_____

_____

_____

_____

_____

_____

_____

_____

_____

_____

_____

_____

Before we move on, here's a question for you: Of the five characters we've been talking about, which one of yours wrote *to* your body
part? Which one *answered?*

Which character wrote? _____

Which character answered? _____

Fern: "No doubt about it. My Problematic Parent wrote and my
Hungry Child answered."

Brendan: "Ditto for me."

Mary: "I came up with the same thing."

What did the exercise put you through emotionally?

Fern: "I don't know why it should surprise me, but it's amazing
how hostile my Problematic Parent was. I picked my thighs, and just
listen to what I wrote."

Fern's Problematic Parent Letter to Her Thighs

Dear Thighs,

You are huge and grotesque, with ugly creases in the fat.
There is absolutely nothing beautiful or graceful or aestheti-

*I am always with myself,
and it is I who am my
tormentor.*

—LEO TOLSTOY

cally pleasing about you. You prevent me from dancing; you even prevent me from walking. I have to hide you and pretend that you aren't part of me and aren't as ugly as you truly are.

You make me a freak.

I hate you.

Fern placed the pencil in her nondominant hand and, in a childish, awkward scrawl, her thighs responded:

Screw you. I am your Frankenstein. You made me what I am. You drove the car that damaged me and now you're upset because the car got dents. Screw you.

Brendan: "I picked my stomach. For such a big stomach, I wrote a small letter."

Brendan's Problematic Parent Letter to His Stomach

To Whom It May Concern:

Go away! Take off. Hit the road, Jack, and don't you come back no more, no more. Stop trying to take over everything.

Brendan placed the pencil in his nondominant hand and, in a childish, awkward scrawl, his stomach responded:

I don't understand why you hate me. If you hadn't been so mean to me, I might have turned out different. Anyway, you'd find something wrong with me no matter what I looked like.

Finally, here's Mary's exchange of letters:

Mary's Problematic Parent Letter to Her Hips

Dear Hips,

What's wrong with you? Have you no shame? No sense of decency? It's time you were cut down to size. You make me sick and tired.

Unfondly,
Mary

I know but one freedom and that is the freedom of the mind.

—ANTOINE DE SAINT-EXUPÉRY

Mary placed the pencil in her nondominant hand and, in a childish, awkward scrawl, her hips responded:

I'm sorry. I did almost everything I was asked. I never asked for much for myself. Besides, you always gave me food as a treat or to quiet me down. So what do you expect of me now?

Hopefully,
Mary

~

Digging for facts is a better mental exercise than jumping to conclusions.

—UNKNOWN

Mary: "What really overwhelmed me about doing this was not the letter from my Problematic Parent, but what I felt answering with the nondominant hand. Using that other hand made me feel so helpless. So childlike."

How about you? Was your Problematic Parent more or less critical than Fern's? How about your response back from *your* body part? Was it more or less defensive than Brendan's? More or less apologetic than Mary's? Did you also *feel* childlike and helpless when you were writing with your nondominant hand?

Let's go back now to the vicious cycle we've been talking about. The *event* here was looking at your body part. Then came your *thoughts,* undoubtedly those from a Problematic Parent. If there was no Adult to be seen, then the Hungry Child, brought out by the nondominant hand, emerged to answer. What follows thoughts, of course, are feelings. What *feelings* did your Hungry Child have?

Fern: "Mine were anger and resentment."
Brendan: "Mine felt defective and ashamed."
Mary: "Unloved. Hurt."

Given those feelings, what *behaviors* might ensue?
Fern: "I'd probably isolate from the world a little more."
Brendan: "I'd probably be circling items in my Big Man catalogue."
Mary: "I'd go right to sleep."

Finally, what are the *consequences* of those behaviors? We all know. Overeating. Every time we live out the script where we come out the Hungry Child, we find ourselves back at square one, in the middle of a binge, eating on automatic pilot. You feel terrible about yourself and the food consolidates and consoles the overwhelming feelings of failure. The cycle is complete. You're back home.

What we're going to do to see if we can break the cycle is take the Problematic Parent and Hungry Child and put them on the stage. I want you to visualize them. It may help to go back to the drawings you did last week.

When you're ready, when your mental stage is set, close your eyes again and watch the curtain rise. Visualize your two characters making their entrance. Imagine them interacting, talking to each other, perhaps with similar dialogue to that which you used in your letters.

As they continue to talk, let your attention slowly shift to a darkened corner of the stage. Standing there is your Adult. Give your Adult an attitude. A voice. A name. Keep giving your Adult features as you imagine it silently observing your version of the Problematic Parent and the Hungry Child.

Now direct your Adult to walk slowly toward the two characters onstage. Have your Adult speak, first to the Problematic Parent. Have the Problematic Parent respond. Get the two of them going at each other. Imagine this really happening. Visualize your Hungry Child standing by, listening to this argument. Write down below what your Hungry Child might hear.

Explore thyself. Herein are demanded the eye and the nerve.

—HENRY DAVID THOREAU

Adult to Problematic Parent	Problematic Parent to Adult
_____	_____
_____	_____
_____	_____
_____	_____

When the exchange is over, close your eyes again and imagine your Adult walking over to your Hungry Child and taking her or his hand. Remember, your Adult is there to provide a reasoned, analytical, problem-solving voice. What does it say to your Hungry Child?

Adult to Hungry Child:

_____

_____

_____

_____

Using your nondominant hand, have your Hungry Child answer the Adult.

Hungry Child to Adult:

_____

_____

_____

_____

After you've finished, close your eyes again. This time I want you to visualize your Hungry Child standing hand in hand with the Adult. Watch them slowly walk off the stage together. Imagine the curtain slowly descending. Focus on the Hungry Child. Look closely.

When Fern brought her Adult into play, here's an abridged version of what she heard:

Fern's Adult: "Take my hand and listen to me. You had me with you in the department store and it worked. I will never let you be hurt like this again. If you're unhappy with your thighs, we can talk about some practical things you could consider doing."

Fern: "When I brought in my Adult, whom I decided to call the Shepherd, I felt that I was okay. That I didn't have to be perfect. That someone would take care of me. I felt hopeful. Hopeful and safe."

Safe and protected is just what you want your Hungry Child to feel. With yourself and with others. The work you did this week is intended to help you begin to develop the tools that will make this happen on a regular basis. I hope this week was a small step in the right direction.

This marks the end of the Discovery stage of the workbook. Like Fern, you will continue to make new discoveries for yourself. Be patient. Subtle changes are happening. _It just takes time._

No one can make you feel inferior without your consent.

—ELEANOR ROOSEVELT

FOOD FOR THOUGHT

WEEK EIGHT

Day One

List those people in your life, living or deceased, who represent a Problematic Parent to you and why.

Person   **Reason**

——————————————— ———————————————

——————————————— ———————————————

——————————————— ———————————————

Day Two

List those people in your life, living or deceased, who represent a Loving Parent to you and why.

Person   **Reason**

——————————————— ———————————————

——————————————— ———————————————

——————————————— ———————————————

Day Three

List those people in your life, living or deceased, who represent an Adult to you and why.

Person   **Reason**

——————————————— ———————————————

——————————————— ———————————————

——————————————— ———————————————

Day Four

List those people in your life, living or deceased, who represent a Nourished Child to you and why.

Person   **Reason**

_____   _____
_____   _____
_____   _____

Day Five

List those people in your life, living or deceased, who represent a Hungry Child to you and why.

Person   **Reason**

_____   _____
_____   _____
_____   _____

Day Six

Take each Problematic Parent you identified in Day One and recall any situation in the past that triggered your Hungry Child.

Problematic Parent   **Situation**

_____   _____
_____   _____
_____   _____

Day Seven

Rewrite each situation using your Adult to intervene.

Situation   **Adult Intervention**

_____   _____
_____   _____
_____   _____

Weekly Checklist

___ 1. Did you complete your Food for Thought writing exercises?

___ 2. Are you using the Eating Awareness Exercise when confronted with trigger foods?

___ 3. Are you using the Vicious Cycle Worksheet to analyze trigger events? See accompanying worksheet.

THE VICIOUS CYCLE WORKSHEET

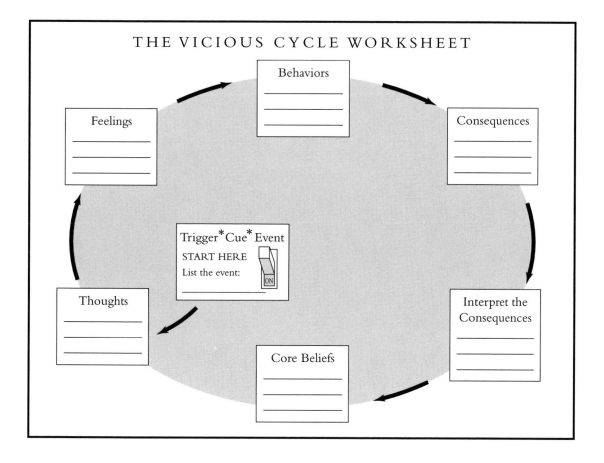

Stage Three

❧

Recovery

The Turning Point

❧

*Get out your binoculars. Train them on your Adult. Observe closely
how when your Adult walks onstage, the play takes an unexpected
turn.*

We now begin the Recovery part of our journey. During the next four
weeks, I am going to ask you to be even more active in working with
the material. I'll be here to help guide you along the way, but you need
to stay focused and push yourself. The more we change, the more our
old selves try to sabotage our efforts. Now is the critical moment to
forge ahead.

Fern: "I do get glimpses of what it feels like to be doing well on
my own, particularly at moments when I have my usual negative
thoughts about myself, and then consciously use what I'm learning
here to fight those thoughts."

Brendan: "I'm proud to say that I've started going to the gym I
joined and I am at least *walking* on the treadmill. So I'm literally being
more *active* these days and it feels like a very basic part of my recovery."

Mary: "For me, I think asking my husband to get *me* a piece of pie
a few weeks ago has been a real turning point. I still can't believe what
a profound effect asking for something had on me. I don't know where
this will take me, but I have the feeling that nothing for me can be

❧

*We have only one shot at
liberation, and that is to
emancipate ourselves from
within.*

—COLETTE DOWLING

quite the same again. It's ironic, of course, that it was my asking for *pie,* of all things, that was such a positive thing for me."

As you can see, things are starting to happen for Fern, Brendan, and Mary. I hope they are for you also. Before we move forward, though, let's take a quick look back and recap what we've accomplished up to this point.

In Weeks One through Four, we learned that the decisions we made about ourselves during our early years formed the basis of our core belief system, how we see and interpret ourselves and the world around us. This belief system came into being before we were old enough to have a fully developed internalized Adult to help us out. Yet until now this old belief system has been what's been propelling us unconsciously and unhappily through life.

The reason for the struggle is that during these early years, we were vulnerable to the verbal and nonverbal messages we received from significant people in our lives. What we've learned in recent weeks is that the unconscious decisions we made about ourselves were exactly that: unconscious. And when the messages we received from others were problematic, the decisions we made about ourselves set up a pattern of behaviors that caused us to crash-land time and time again.

Getting in touch with those patterns and discovering that we do, indeed, have a fully functioning Adult available to us now doesn't mean we always use it, any more than we might take advantage of our physical potential or other resources. When we banish the Adult from our emotional landscape, we propel ourselves back into our old script. We are back in the vicious cycle we've been talking about the last four weeks. It's in this vicious cycle that we see the old script being played out by the characters in our head who drive our compulsive eating behaviors. The compulsive eating, in turn, takes us back to those very thoughts and feelings about ourselves that validate our core belief system.

And what's going on, as we discovered in the last couple of weeks, is that the tired old script with the unhappy ending depends on an interaction between two featured players: the Problematic Parent and the Hungry Child. Our goal now is give that Adult a far stronger role in the script so that it can effectively challenge the messages generated by the Problematic Parent. To *exercise* the Adult, then, is to *exorcise* the Problematic Parent.

A riot is at bottom the language of the unheard.

—MARTIN LUTHER KING, JR.

To begin, I will be asking you to participate in a visualization exercise. As the Adult, you will be asked to imagine that you have the power to bring your Problematic Parent to life. He or she will be seated in a large chair across from you, and you will have an opportunity to speak to him or her. But first, before you begin, let's see how Brendan's dialogue went.

Brendan's Adult to his Problematic Parent: "It's taken a long time, but I'm finally starting to get you off my back. I'm a big boy now. I no longer have to subject myself to your abuse. I'm independent. I'm successful. I don't need to look to you for anything. I can look to others and myself for support when I need it."

Brendan's Problematic Parent replies: "You're very funny, kid. Successful? To who? Not to me. Never were and never will be. Last time I checked, you had no wife or family. And your so-called career? Gambling with other people's money? At least I worked honestly, with my hands. So stop being so high-and-mighty. If it weren't for me, you wouldn't be here. And trust me, you're going to miss me when I'm gone."

Brendan's Adult responds: "Thank you for helping to make me. Thank you for those qualities I inherited from you, especially my humor, which I value. As for the rest of what you said, I know that is coming from your alcoholism. It's the booze speaking, and I refuse to take it personally. So lots of luck, wherever you are. And when we meet again, I hope it's in a place that doesn't serve bourbon."

All serious daring starts from within.

—EUDORA WELTY

Brendan's reaction to this exercise? "When I finally got into this, it was very powerful. It's not so much that my adult clearly carried the day, but it did give me a feeling of . . . power is the word that keeps coming to mind, that I don't usually have. I will tell you honestly that there was also a little part of me waiting to get hit."

Of course there was. Good change takes time. Now let's see where this dialogue took Mary.

Mary's Adult to her Problematic Parent: "I have spent my whole life acting like everything was okay, that it was my job to take care of everyone else. This I learned from you, and now I am struggling to unlearn it. I no longer have to take the blame when things don't go right. I can be a good person and still have needs. Saint Mary is going to take early retirement."

Mary's Problematic Parent replies: "Stop your complaining. You had a roof over your head and a warm meal in your stomach every night. You should be counting your blessings instead of blaming me."

Mary's Adult responds: "I don't mean to blame you. I do thank you for meeting my physical needs. But for the first time, I'm being honest, especially with myself. You were unavailable and incapable of meeting my emotional needs. I have no trouble finding forgiveness in my heart, because I know you did the best you could. But I need to say that I was left feeling alone, lost, empty, dependent on food for emotional nourishment. That's what I'm dealing with now."

Mary's thoughts about this exchange? "It's fascinating what this exercise put me through. Part of me felt exhilarated saying the things that my Adult said. But I have to admit that when I replied to my Problematic Parent, I really had to fight feeling guilty. I don't know if I can ever get over feeling guilty."

Maybe not. But I think it's important for Mary and all of us to know that the goal of this exercise and any other ones we do is not to trash our parents or anyone else, living or dead. It's to get in touch with our own thoughts and feelings, to be unafraid to express them. Fear. Guilt. These are among the barriers that have kept us away from ourselves in the past. Mary, in fact, could look to her own religion for supportive words: "Ye shall know the truth and the truth shall set ye free."

Time now for Fern's role-playing.

Fern's Adult to her Problematic Parent: "Dear Perfect Person, I am, in every sense of the expression, fed up with your depressing righteousness. Why don't you give us both a break and ease up on the negative feedback. You must be aware that after all these years, whatever you're trying to accomplish isn't working. Not for either of us. Your opinions. Your judgments. All the things you seem to want for me. They're your things, not mine. I have to keep telling myself that. I need an emotional divorce from you."

Fern's Problematic Parent replies: "You're so emotional. You ought to go back on that medication you used to take for whatever that thing you had was, except it made you gain weight. Maybe if you had a clearer head you would understand how much I care about you. After all, if I don't kick you in the ass about your appearance, who will? It's because I love you and I know you'll never get a man looking the way you do. Trust me. I'm your mother. P.S. I'm very proud to have a daugh-

Don't hug your defeats. Analyze your victories.

—UNKNOWN

ter who's a lawyer. You could ask any of my friends. I brag about you all the time."

Fern's Adult responds: "I can see I'm wasting my time. You don't have a clue. It's hard for me to accept, but you're not going to change. I guess that means change will have to come from me. Maybe I just need to forgive myself for not being the daughter you think you wanted and get on with it. I think rebelling against you has been as bad for me as doing it your way. P.S. When you brag about me to your friends, that's not love. Trust *me*."

How did all this sit with Fern? "Stepping back and looking at what I wrote as the Adult, I think I didn't really have the right voice. I just couldn't drop the sarcasm and anger that I usually have. Maybe I should go back and rewrite it so it's calmer, but *not* because of what my mother said about my being emotional. I would have to do it for me."

Now it's your turn. Take out a pencil or pen and, speaking in *your* Adult voice, use the space below to write whatever you'd like to say to *your* Problematic Parent. Remember your Adult is rational, analytical, problem-solving.

My Adult to My Problematic Parent

_____

_____

_____

_____

Now imagine yourself getting up, walking over to the Problematic Parent's chair, and sitting down in it. In that role, have your Problematic Parent respond.

My Problematic Parent to My Adult

_____

_____

_____

_____

When you have duly arranged your "facts" in logical order, lo, it is like an oil lamp that you have made, filled and trimmed, but which sheds no light unless first you light it.

—ANTOINE DE SAINT-EXUPÉRY

Finally, switch chairs again and see what your Adult has to say by way of response to your Problematic Parent.

My Adult to My Problematic Parent

_____

_____

_____

_____

Take a moment to reflect. What kinds of thoughts and feelings do you have about the dialogue you just created?

Let's move on now to the next visualization exercise. In this one, you will be asked to imagine your Adult in one chair and your Hungry Child in the other. Again, let's first see how this exchange went for Fern, Brendan, and Mary.

Fern's Adult to her Hungry Child: "I understand why you are angry. You have been deprived of a voice for a long time. Now I am here to listen. I realize how insensitive, controlling, and cruel your mother can be. I know how desperately you miss your dad. You can scream. You have a right to feel hurt and angry. I am only sorry that it takes such a toll on you. Together, maybe we can find a better way."

Fern's Hungry Child answers: "What you say makes sense in my head. It's all there clear as a bell, but when it comes to 'letting go' and breaking old patterns, it's so hard. Everything needs to be translated— 'Problematic Parent . . . Loving Parent . . . Adult'—it's like learning a new language."

Fern's Adult: "Yes it is, and just think about it. Could it be any other way? Look at how far you've come already from when you would scream and bang your head against the wall for hours. I'm proud of you. If you keep practicing, it will get easier. And remember. I'm on twenty-four-hour call. Reach out for me, anytime, day or night."

Fern's reaction to her writings: "It's reassuring. I only hope I can keep that Adult alive in me."

Next comes Mary.

Mary's Adult to her Hungry Child: "Peek-a-boo, I see you! Why are you hiding? Are you sad? Are you scared? Are you angry or are we

Facts do not cease to exist because they are ignored.

—ALDOUS HUXLEY

playing a game? If it's a game, please tell me the rules so I can play, too. I'd like to play with you. If you are upset, won't you tell me why? If I know the reason, maybe I can help make it better."

Mary's Hungry Child: "Go away! No, stay. I want you to stay, but I feel funny when you look at me. So don't look at me. But stay and talk to me."

Mary's Adult replies: "I would be happy to stay and talk with you. If you don't want me to look at you, of course I won't. But when you're ready, I would like to know why you feel funny when I look at you. I want you to know that I like what I see. I see a pretty, smart, strong little girl with a big heart. I see someone who is generous and kind. Does it bother you that I see these things? That I am here to protect you?"

Mary's reaction to what she's written: "Overwhelmed. Hearing these words from my Adult is almost too much. It's going to take me time to get used to this kind of attention."

Listen now to Brendan.

Brendan's Adult to his Hungry Child: "I know I haven't been around much for you over the years, but I hope better late than never. I want you to know that I understand why you have spent so much of your life trying to be liked and loved. I also want you to know how much I love your humor, and although you use it often to protect yourself, that doesn't mean you have to discard it. My only concern is that in trying to be the life of the party, you have used food and alcohol and drugs and have put your interests and your health in jeopardy. I'm here to help you change that."

Brendan's Hungry Child: "Thanks. I need all the help I can get. I still don't fully understand why it's so important to put a smile on everyone else's face at my own expense. If you will protect me from you-know-who and help me get control of this once and for all, I will be more grateful than you'll ever know. I'll even buy you a free membership in my health club."

Brendan's Adult: "Very funny. Okay, I accept. I'll meet you by the Stairmaster."

Brendan's reaction: "Relief. I like the idea that my Adult can have a sense of humor."

Once again, it's your turn. With your pen in hand, create a dialogue between *your* Adult and Hungry Child.

*Reason can wrestle
And overthrow terror.*

—EURIPIDES

My Adult to My Hungry Child

_____
_____
_____

The reply:

My Hungry Child to My Adult

_____
_____
_____
_____

And finally, the last word from your Adult:

My Adult to My Hungry Child

_____
_____
_____
_____

Spend a few minutes now going back over what you've just written. Let the words sink in. What kinds of thoughts do you have? What kinds of feelings? Take your time before moving on.

Okay, if you're finished reflecting on your Adult and Hungry Child, it's time to play musical chairs again. This time we have the Adult and Loving Parent exchanging words.

Let's look at the words Fern had with her Loving Parent.

Fern's Adult to her Loving Parent: "Dad, I really miss you. I know that Richie was probably your favorite, but I know you loved me, too. You always seemed to accept me for who I was. Those magical moments late at night when we'd raid the refrigerator together and try to stifle our giggles as we stood there in the dark are still as vivid as if it was yesterday. I know I need to let go of that part of our relationship, but it's hard."

Fern's Loving Parent: "I'm never far away from you, sweetheart.

The mind is its own place, and in itself can make a heav'n of hell, a hell of heav'n.

—JOHN MILTON

Just reach out and I'll be there. My only hope is that you use the memories you have of us to help yourself, not hurt yourself. I love you."

Fern's Adult: "I love you, too. I'll try to keep you with me in the best possible ways."

Fern's reaction: "Tearful!"

Fern's reaction to this exercise was very powerful and will definitely provide the impetus she needs to move herself forward in the weeks to come.

Now it's your turn. Sitting across from your Adult is your Loving Parent. Talk to her or him.

My Adult to My Loving Parent

_____

_____

_____

_____

My Loving Parent to My Adult

_____

_____

_____

_____

My Adult to My Loving Parent

_____

_____

_____

_____

❧

We should not let our fears hold us back from pursuing our hopes.

—JOHN F. KENNEDY

Last but not least, let's bring to life the Nourished Child. Seat her or him in front of you to have a little talk. Again, before we proceed, let's see what Mary came up with.

Mary's Adult to the Nourished Child: "Wake up, little one. I know you have been sound asleep for a long time. But now I am here to give you what you've been starving for all your life."

Mary's Nourished Child: "What will it be like if I wake up? Can I run and play and have fun?"

Mary's Adult: "You can do what you want to do. You will become what you were always meant to be. In your life story, it's time for the ugly duckling to turn into the swan. And I'll always be by your side to make sure you're okay."

Now it's time for you to talk with your Nourished Child.

My Adult to My Nourished Child

_____

_____

_____

_____

My Nourished Child to My Adult

∾

Adopt the pace of nature.
Her secret is patience.

—RALPH WALDO EMERSON

_____

_____

_____

_____

My Adult to My Nourished Child

_____

_____

_____

_____

Mary observed that she liked her Adult voice. This realization is a very important one. No one of us has the *same* adult voice, yet each of us must be *comfortable* with our Adult voice, especially if we are to use it effectively in the presence of our Problematic Parent. Problematic Parents can run over us like a tank or snipe at us like a mosquito. To disarm them, our Adult can take the form of an antitank missile or a flyswatter. All that matters is that what we bring into play is a part of our emotional arsenal we feel good about using.

Bringing that Adult voice into play is scary because very few people are attracted to conflict, and many people will respond defensively, angrily, to what your Adult has to say. If it's any comfort, let me reassure you that when you lose your voice in a relationship with a Problematic Parent figure, when your Hungry Child retreats into food, *the conflict is still there.* Between Fern and the car dealer. Brendan and his father. Mary and her supervisor.

As Fern, Brendan, and Mary developed their Adult voices, here's what they discovered:

Fern: "My Adult doesn't work when I stare at someone in anger. It's best when I use my skills as a lawyer. I try to imagine I have that person on the witness stand, and I'm asking lots of questions. 'Did I hear you say that . . .' or 'Was it your intent . . .' Questions like that seem to throw the other person, and I'm starting to realize that I don't really care what the other person's intent was. I just want them to stop acting like a Problematic Parent, and this method seems to really work for me."

Brendan: "A technique that I've begun to experiment with involves changing the subject. When I was a kid, I would try to do that with my old man when he was on my case. He would be yelling about whatever, and if I said something like 'Hey, the Celtics won tonight!' he might back off. Then I was afraid. Now I use that tactic to take charge. An example was when I went to sign up for a dating service and the woman who ran it kept pushing to know how much money I earned. She already had enough information about me to know I make a decent living, but she really wanted exact amounts. I asked why this was relevant, and she said many women she represented thought this was very important. So I just said, 'I'm sure they do. Could you tell me a little more now about your fee and how many members you have and how your service works?' My changing the subject was really effective here because she stopped asking about my income."

Mary: "Like Fern and Brendan, what's working for me is taking something I'm already familiar with that I've always used at my own expense and turning it around for my benefit. For me, that's being nice. I know I do nice well. So what my Adult seems to be emerging as is someone who approaches conflict in the nicest possible way. It really helps me when I say things like 'I don't mean to be impolite, but . . .' or 'If you'll forgive me for saying this . . .' I'm doing this with my supervisor at work lately. Every time she opens her trap, I look at her politely and cock my head and say, 'I beg your pardon?' It hasn't turned her completely around, but it definitely makes *me* feel better."

Only in growth, reform and change, paradoxically enough, is true security found.

—ANNE MORROW LINDBERGH

༈

How about you? What does your Adult voice sound like? Think about that now and practice with it whenever you can. You may even want to do it standing in front of a mirror so that you can become comfortable not only with your Adult's voice but with its facial expressions and body language.

I hope the role-playing, dialogues, and visualizations you've just completed, along with reading what Fern, Brendan, and Mary wrote, has been helpful to you. I've designed these expressive exercises, along with those elsewhere in the workbook, specifically to increase your immediate awareness of feelings, perceptions, and sensations; that is, your in-the-moment experience. This approach can facilitate the uncovering of buried feelings and memories. It also can be very useful in helping your Adult become aware of, understand, take charge of, and integrate your "internal family." This chapter, then, provides the cornerstone for the recovery phase of *The Hunger Within* and for all the material we'll be covering in the weeks to come.

The daily Food for Thought exercises that follow are designed to help your Adult begin to modify your script with the real people in your life today. Please take the time to complete them before moving on to Week Ten.

FOOD FOR THOUGHT

WEEK NINE

Day One

Of the Problematic Parent figures in your life today that you first identified in Week Seven, pick the biggest one. As the Adult, take that person through the visualization and writing exercise you did this week.

My Adult to _____:

_____

_____

_____

_____

The fearful unbelief is unbelief in yourself.

—THOMAS CARLYLE

_____ to My Adult:

_____

_____

_____

_____

My Adult to _____:

_____

_____

_____

_____

Day Two

Read the following brief scenario and let your Adult respond accordingly:

When I express a concern I have about something to someone in my family, that person "discounts" me by not listening or telling me not to worry about it or whatever. Here's how my Adult can protect me in this situation:

_____

_____

_____

_____

Day Three

Read the following brief scenario and let your Adult respond accordingly:

I learn that a coworker (neighbor, if you don't work) has spread an unflattering piece of gossip about me. Whether or not it's true, my Adult can protect me by:

_____

_____

_____

_____

Our greatest glory is not in never failing, but in rising every time we fall.

—UNKNOWN

Day Four

Read the following brief scenario and let your Adult respond accordingly:

At a dinner party, my hostess, who knows I'm being careful about what I eat, keeps trying to foist fattening foods on me and implies that I'm being somehow rude if I don't try her goose liver. My Adult can get me out of this predicament by:

_____
_____
_____
_____

Day Five

You know that it is the Problematic Parent messages inside your own head and from the outside world that fuel your Hungry Child and compulsive eating. Identify specific ways your Adult can help your Hungry Child head off "trigger switches" at the pass in the following three situations:

When I am home, my Adult will _____

_____

When I am at work, my Adult will _____

_____

When I am in social situations, my Adult will _____

_____

Day Six

If you find that the "trigger" has been pulled and the Hungry Child has taken over center stage, list the strategies your Adult can bring to bear to circumvent the vicious cycle in the following arenas:

When I am home, my Adult can _____

_____

When I am at work, my Adult can _____

_____

When I am in social situations, my Adult can _____

_____

Day Seven

If you find that you fell back into your old script and played it out to the bitter end, to a binge, call on your Adult to analyze the situation.

    1. Identify the event or situation that activated your script.

    _____

    _____

    2. Using the Vicious Cycle Worksheet in Week Five, track the steps you went through to come to a miserable conclusion about yourself. See the accompanying worksheet.

    Thoughts: _____

    _____

    Feelings: _____

    _____

    Behaviors: _____

    _____

    Consequences: _____

    _____

    3. Bring your Adult to life now. Since your Adult knows that the script you played out brings you "back home," have it help you understand why in this situation, you needed to revisit your old haunts.

    _____

    _____

Weekly Checklist

___ 1. Did you complete the visualization and writing exercises in this chapter?

___ 2. Did you complete the Food for Thought writing exercises?

THE VICIOUS CYCLE WORKSHEET

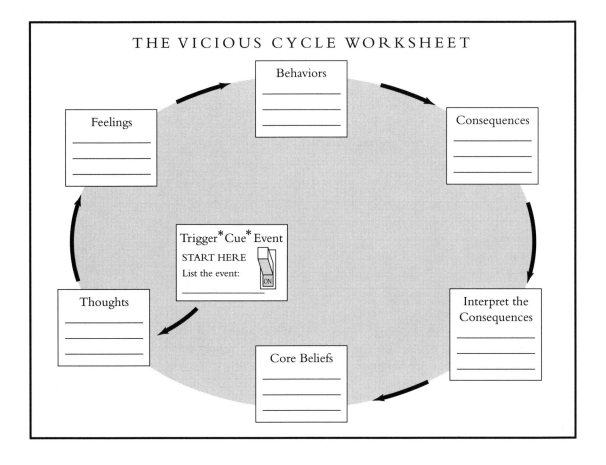

Back to the Future

❧

I think one must finally take one's life in one's arms.
—Arthur Miller, *After the Fall*

Taking your life in your arms is precisely what you'll be doing this week. By listening to the gentle whispers within yourself, you will continue on your inner journey toward recovery. You will get closer to an inner peace. To a sense of well-being. To a feeling of security.

Way back in Week One, we talked about the functions obsessive thoughts and compulsive behaviors serve for us. How they offer us an escape from feelings that our Hungry Child can't handle. How they were originally an adaptive coping mechanism because we had no internalized Adult to help us out. How our obsessions and compulsions disconnected us from the world around us and, more important, from ourselves.

Now is the time to get *reconnected*.

The emphasis last week was on your Adult. This week we are going to encourage this reconnection, this reunion with ourselves, by accessing the most vulnerable part of who we are. Our Adult will be with us all the way. So will someone else.

You know the old cliché "A picture is worth a thousand words." For what we're about to do, I think it's worth a lot more. What I'd like

❧
Everything intercepts us from ourselves.

—RALPH WALDO EMERSON

for you to do now is get out the scrapbooks or rummage through the drawers or attic or call a relative. I want you to do whatever you can to find a photograph of yourself. Preferably as a child between the ages of two and six—toddler to early elementary school. If you have a choice, pick a photo that you are particularly fond of, that you feel particularly close to, that elicits any strong feelings, good or bad. If you absolutely can't lay your hands on a photo, you can use the Hungry Child drawing of yourself you made in Week Seven, or you can close your eyes and try to imagine a picture of yourself when you were young.

Okay. Now get that photo!

Before you begin the upcoming visualization exercise, I'm going to give you a sneak preview by showing you what this experience was like for Brendan. First I asked Brendan to imagine the child pictured in his photo coming to life and seated next to him. Then I asked him to take the child by the hand and start a dialogue. Brendan began the dialogue by writing a letter to the child in his photo. The child was then asked to respond using his nondominant hand. Here's what evolved:

Brendan's Letter to His Child

Dear Little One,

I had forgotten what a great little kid you were, and what a tough road you had to travel. Hey, cheer up. You're a survivor. That was then and this is now. God, I wish I could have done something for you all those years. I look at you and I know who you are. I really do. And now I'm here and we're both safe. Here's looking at you, kid.

Brendan's Child Responds

Dear Grown Up Brendan,

Where have you been? I had almost given up on you. I was always there, but where were you? How could you forget me? So now you show up. But how do I know you are who you say you are? How do I really know?

Brendan's reaction: "The letters had meaning for me, but they

---

One ought to hold on to one's heart; for if one lets it go, one soon loses control of the head too.

—Friedrich Wilhelm Nietzsche

didn't begin to capture the feelings I had when I looked at my picture and then closed my eyes. I felt such pain. That little boy was so unprotected. There was no one there for him. And then when I was supposed to take his hand, that was very hard also. The little boy was afraid to let *anyone* take his hand. When it happened in my fantasy, when the hands touched, it was almost too much. Maybe that's why my child's response was pretty guarded."

Ready to give it a shot? All right, before we begin this exercise, I'd like to urge you not to stop if you find yourself feeling awkward or embarrassed. These feelings are usually the first sign that you're "reconnecting" with yourself, something that may feel very unfamiliar to you.

Place your photo in front of you. Study it carefully. Take your time. Now close your eyes and imagine the child in the photo coming to life. She or he is sitting next to you. Picture yourself taking the child by the hand. You have the opportunity at this moment to say anything in the world to this child. With your eyes still closed, spend as long as you'd like thinking about what that will be. When you know, open your eyes and write your words down in the space below.

As is our confidence, so is our capacity.
—WILLIAM HAZLITT

To My Child

_____

_____

_____

_____

If what you just finished was a casual experience, I'd like to suggest that you go back and look at the photo again. See if you can let down your guard enough to ease into the picture, to let the reconnection happen. Then close your eyes again and give it another shot.

What I'd like you to do next is to use a technique that we introduced in Week Eight when we dialogued with a body part using our nondominant hand. This time, close your eyes again and imagine that you are now the child in the photo, the child that you were. This child has just heard what you had to say. Imagine how it might respond. When you have an idea, open your eyes and, using your nondominant hand, write the child's response in the space below.

My Child to Me

_____

_____

_____

_____

What was this exchange like for you? What were your thoughts and feelings? Write them here.

_____

_____

_____

_____

Now let's take a look at how this exercise went for Mary and Fern.

Mary to Her Child

Dear Mary,

You look so lovable. I just want to hug you and not let you go. I want to put you in my pocket and carry you around with me everywhere I go and never leave you alone. I want to hear everything you have to say. I want to know what you're thinking and feeling. I want to play with you. But most of all I want to hug you and kiss you and never stop!

Love, Me

Mary's Child

Dear Me,

Hooray, my very own grown up. I want you all to myself. I always felt all my brothers and sisters got you. I don't want to share you now with anyone. How do I know you will always love me? Do I have to look lovable to be loved? Will you promise not to go away?

Mary's reaction: "My child sure seems to be starving for attention. Her words are certainly those of a Hungry Child. Like Brendan's Child, you can read between the lines and hear the distrust, the fear of aban-

Self-esteem isn't everything, it's just that there's nothing without it.

—GLORIA STEINEM

donment. Also like Brendan, really looking at the photo of me was very powerful. It's not so much what I saw as what I didn't see. I look at that little girl and it's like she's not there. She has this nice little dress and this blank look on her face and it's like she's invisible. My pain comes thinking about it now because it really hits home that she *was* invisible."

Fern to Her Child

When I look at you, sweetheart, my heart fills with love and I want to gather you up in a long, warm hug. I want to touch your soft skin and hold your tiny hand and skip with you, sing to you, laugh with you in the sunshine. I love your big smile. I love your funny crooked pigtails. I miss you, baby. I'm so sorry that I lost you. I really am.

Fern's Child

I'm sorry too. I thought I had forgotten about hugs and songs and sweetheart. Knowing that it's still there, that I still want these things, is hard for me to accept. You buried me Alive!!! I lost You!!! And I'm not sure about you now. I want you. I don't want you. I want you. I don't want you. I want you. I don't want you. I want you. I don't want you.

Fern's reaction: "My child sounds suspicious and angry. I think her anger runs very deep. On the other hand, there is that other side of her, I guess, that wants to believe what's being said to her. One thing is certain. It's not going to be easy to get her out of her black hole."

No, it's not. Not for Fern. Not for Brendan. Not for Mary. The letters written with the dominant hand were for the most part those of a Loving Parent. The responses from the children were characterized by confusion, doubt, caution, and/or anger. Was that equally true for your Child's letter? Was your Child something less than eager to accept the loving gifts being offered?

If your Child did not jump to embrace you, that's because there was so much hunger in your Child. And with good reason. The Child that can proceed confidently, trusting itself and its environment, is the Nourished Child. For the Hungry Child, trust does not come easily.

*Ah, great it is to believe
As we stand in youth by
the starry stream;
But a great thing is to
fight life through,
And at the end, "The
dream is true!"*

—EDWIN MARKHAM

If this sounds pessimistic, I certainly don't mean it to be. Quite the opposite. Your Adult can and will help your Nourished Child emerge. One way you can do this is by taking an analytical look at the letters you have written and sorting out exactly who is saying what. Using the Letter-Writing Analysis Worksheet that you'll be filling out later, I asked Brendan, Mary, and Fern to go back to their letters and break them down line by line. In the letters written to the Child in the photo, I wanted to know which phrases were *strokes*, coming from their Loving Parent, which were *put-downs* coming from their Problematic Parent. In the Child's responses, I asked them to identify which words were *positive interpretations* coming from the mouth of their Nourished Child, which words were *negative interpretations* coming from their Hungry Child. Finally, I asked them to use the elements in the vicious cycle to track where all this led.

Let's see how their worksheets look:

BRENDAN'S WORKSHEET

Letter to the Child

LOVING PARENT (STROKES)	PROBLEMATIC PARENT (PUT-DOWNS)
Great little kid	I had forgotten
I know who you are	Cheer up (for some reason, sounds like a put-down)
I'm here and we're both safe	That was then and this is now (I'm not sure whether this is LP or PP)

Child's Responses

NOURISHED CHILD (positive interpretations)	HUNGRY CHILD (negative interpretations)
I had almost given up on you	Where have you been?
	Where were you?
	How could you forget me?
	So now you show up.
	How do I know you are who you say you are?

FEELINGS	FEELINGS
(created by positive thoughts)	(created by negative thoughts)
Slight amount of hope	Sad
	Untrusting
	Longing
	Pissed

LIKELY BEHAVIORS	LIKELY BEHAVIORS
(created by positive thoughts)	(created by negative feelings)
Hopefully less food, more feelings	Round up all the usual suspects.
	Watch TV
	Use humor to help me hide.
	Retreat into food
	(I know I can trust it)

CONSEQUENCES	CONSEQUENCES
(anticipated outcome)	(anticipated outcome)
Not really sure	End up where I started. Lonely and feeling like you-know-what about myself

Brendan's letter provided a series of mixed messages. A few strokes in conjunction with a few put-downs. This verbal exchange fueled a predominantly negative child interpretation, and paints a picture of an untrusting, sad, and angry Hungry Child for Brendan's Adult to analyze.

Now let's take a look at Mary's worksheet.

What things soever ye desire, when ye pray, believe that ye receive them, and ye shall have them.

—MARK 11:24

MARY'S WORKSHEET

Letter to the Child

LOVING PARENT (STROKES)	PROBLEMATIC PARENT (PUT-DOWNS)
You look so lovable	None
I just want to hug you . . .	
Not let you go . . . carry you . . .	
I want to hear . . . I want to know	
hug . . . kiss . . . never stop!	

Child Responses

NOURISHED CHILD	HUNGRY CHILD
(positive interpretations)	(negative interpretations)
I have my very own grown-up	Do I have to look lovable to be lovable?
	My brothers and sisters got all the attention.
	How do I know you'll always love me?
	Promise not to go away.

FEELINGS	FEELINGS
(created by positive thoughts)	(created by negative thoughts)
Excitement	Uncertainty
	Fear
	Neglected
	Disconnected

LIKELY BEHAVIORS	LIKELY BEHAVIORS
(created by positive feelings)	(created by negative feelings)
Smile (not sure if big or small)	Keep being the provider
Take the hand	Withdraw into myself
Do something active (find a swing?)	Eat to fill the void

CONSEQUENCES	CONSEQUENCES
(anticipated outcome)	(anticipated outcome)
A step in the right direction.	Same old stuff. Mary but not merry.
Feel more alive. Better about myself.	

If you compare Brendan and Mary's worksheets, you'll see that although Mary's letter to her Child is filled with many more strokes, the presence of her Hungry Child produces just as many negative interpretations. Here we see a glimmer of the Nourished Child, but it quickly becomes tarnished by the more predominant Hungry Child. A Hungry Child who quickly interprets any kind of stroking in a *nega-*

tive light in attempts to maintain and validate her internalized belief system.

To see an extreme example of how strokes can get you nowhere when your Hungry Child is center stage, study what Fern learned when her Adult did its analysis:

FERN'S WORKSHEET

Letter to the Child

LOVING PARENT (STROKES)	PROBLEMATIC PARENT (PUT-DOWNS)
When I look at you, sweetheart, my heart fills with love. . . . I want to gather you up . . . hug . . . hold . . . skip . . . sing . . . laugh . . . I love your big smile . . . funny pigtails. I miss you. . . . I'm sorry I lost you.	None

Child Responses

NOURISHED CHILD (positive interpretations)	HUNGRY CHILD (negative interpretations)
I still want those things. I still want you.	I'm sorry too Thought I had forgotten Hard for me to accept You buried me ALIVE!!! I lost YOU!!! Not sure about you I don't want you

FEELINGS (created by positive thoughts)	FEELINGS (created by negative thoughts)
Pain (this must mean NC thoughts are really HC thoughts?!)	Angry, Angry, Angry Deprived, bitter Sad Suspicious, cynical

We know what we are, but know not what we may be.

—WILLIAM SHAKESPEARE

Reach high, for stars lie
hidden in your soul.
Dream deep, for every
dream precedes the goal.

—PAMELA VAULL STARR

LIKELY BEHAVIORS
(created by positive feelings)
If pain above is HC feelings,
then I don't have a clue.

LIKELY BEHAVIORS
(created by positive feelings)
Temper tantrums
Work more at the office
Cut off from people
Bakery, here I come

CONSEQUENCES
(anticipated outcome)
For the answer to this, please
contact my HC.

CONSEQUENCES
(anticipated outcome)
You *know* the answer. I don't
even want to write it down.

Once again, a stroking letter resulting in a *negative* child interpretation. Fern's Adult sees a picture of a very angry and suspicious Hungry Child.

Now it's your turn. Using the Letter-Writing Analysis Worksheet that follows, let your Adult analyze your dialogue with the Child in your photo.

LETTER-WRITING ANALYSIS WORKSHEET

Letter to the Child

Loving Parent (strokes)	Problematic Parent (put-downs)
1.	1.
2.	2.
3.	3.
4.	4.
5.	5.

Child Interpretations

Nourished Child	Hungry Child
Thoughts (positive interpretations)	Thoughts (negative interpretations)
1.	1.
2.	2.
3.	3.
4.	4.
5.	5.
Feelings (created by + thoughts)	Feelings (created by − thoughts)
1.	1.
2.	2.
3.	3.
4.	4.
5.	5.
Behaviors (reaction to + feelings)	Behaviors (reaction to − feelings)
1.	1.
2.	2.
3.	3.
4.	4.
5.	5.
Consequences (anticipated outcome)	Consequences (anticipated outcome)
1.	1.
2.	2.
3.	3.
4.	4.
5.	5.

If you've finished filling in your worksheet, I'd like you to go back and read the exchange of letters you had with the Child in your photograph. Using a combination of your Adult and Loving Parent, focus on the Child's interpretations, feelings, behaviors, and consequences. Imagine the Child in your photo experiencing all these things.

Now take a long look at your picture. Then close your eyes and visualize the Child in your photo sitting in front of you. Bringing to bear everything you have learned from the previous exercise, rewrite a letter to her or him in the space below:

Dear _____,

_____

_____

_____

_____

Done? Okay, now place your pencil or pen in your nondominant hand and have your Child respond: _____

_____

_____

_____

_____

One can never consent to creep when one feels an impulse to soar.

—HELEN KELLER

After you have responded, use your dominant hand to answer the Child: _____

_____

_____

_____

_____

In the space below, continue with the dialogue, using the dual-handed technique, until you reach some kind of peace between the two writers. As in any good experience with conflict resolution, you have to stay with it.

To My Child: _____

_____

From My Child: _____

_____

To My Child: _____

_____

From My Child: _____   ❧

_____   *Hope is the feeling you*

To My Child: _____   *have that the feeling you*

_____   *have isn't permanent.*

From My Child: _____   —JEAN KERR

_____

When you have developed a relationship between yourself and the Child in your photograph that is comfortable in the best sense of the word, fill in a new Letter-Writing Analysis Worksheet and see if and how it's different from your first one.

LETTER-WRITING ANALYSIS WORKSHEET

Letter to the Child

Loving Parent (strokes)	*Problematic Parent (put-downs)*
1.	1.
2.	2.
3.	3.
4.	4.
5.	5.

Child Responses

Nourished Child	*Hungry Child*
Thoughts (positive interpretations)	*Thoughts (negative interpretations)*
1.	1.
2.	2.
3.	3.
4.	4.
5.	5.
Feelings (created by + thoughts)	*Feelings (created by - thoughts)*
1.	1.
2.	2.
3.	3.
4.	4.
5.	5.
Behaviors (reaction to + feelings)	*Behaviors (reaction to - feelings)*
1.	1.
2.	2.
3.	3.
4.	4.
5.	5.
Consequences (anticipated outcome)	*Consequences (anticipated outcome)*
1.	1.
2.	2.
3.	3.
4.	4.
5.	5.

Of the rewrites that Fern, Brendan, and Mary did, let me show you Fern's here because her original exchange of letters was so intensely negative.

Fern's rewrite letter to her Child:

Sweetheart,

I want you to know how much I wish I could help you feel the preciousness that is you. I want to take you by the hand and let the safety and love I possess seep into your heart and soul. I think of holding you and hugging you and of you resting your head on my shoulder. I am there for you whenever you need me. I know that beneath your anger you are hurt. You are innocent. You are a gentle little person still waiting to discover the world. I know these things, sweetheart, and I know why you are so guarded with me. I *did* bury you in the past. I stuffed down your words and feelings with food. Now I'm learning how to give you what you need. I know I have to walk the walk before you can trust me. Take all the time you need.

Fern's Child replies:

I really would like to believe what you say. I would like to feel safe with you. But you're right. Talk is cheap. How do I know? How do I know?

Fern to her Child: You don't know. You'd be crazy if you trusted me before I earned it. This is going to take a lot of time, honey. I know that.

Fern's Child: *So what do you want of me? What am I supposed to do now?*

Fern to her Child: Whatever you want. Say what you want. Feel what you want. Be who you want to be. My only hope is that you'll leave the door open for me. That you won't forget I'm here.

Fern's Child: *I'm not making any promises, but I'll try. Just don't expect too much of me.*

Fern to her Child: If you don't completely disconnect from me, that will be enough.

Fern's Child: *I'm not hanging up.*

Life loves to be taken by the lapel and told: "I am with you kid. Let's go."

—MAYA ANGELOU

When Fern's Adult took this exchange of letters and put it into her worksheet, here's what emerged:

FERN'S WORKSHEET

Letter to the Child

LOVING PARENT (STROKES)	PROBLEMATIC PARENT (PUT-DOWNS)
Preciousness, help, safety	None that I know of
Hold, hug, shoulder	
You are hurt	
Innocent, gentle, little person	
Sweetheart	
Take all the time you need	
Feel what you feel	
That will be enough	

Child Responses

NOURISHED CHILD	HUNGRY CHILD
(positive interpretations)	(negative interpretations)
I really would like to believe	Talk is cheap. How do I know?
I'm not hanging up	I'll try
	What do you want of me?
	Don't expect too much of me

FEELINGS	FEELINGS
(created by thoughts)	(created by thoughts)
Less anger (if less of something is something)	Cautious
A ray of hope	Scared
Some actual warmth (let's not get carried away)	Still some anger

LIKELY BEHAVIORS	LIKELY BEHAVIORS
(reaction to positive feelings)	(reaction to negative feelings)
A little more open	Quickly close down again
Maybe I'll take a nice walk	Back to the bakery

CONSEQUENCES
(anticipated outcome)
Okay, I'll admit it. I might feel
a little better about myself

CONSEQUENCES
(anticipated outcome)
My mother will have plenty
to talk about

I hope it's clear to you after looking at Fern's rewrites and her worksheet that although her Hungry Child is less intensely negative, it is still very much there. This time we see glimmers of a Nourished Child, but even they are dotted with a sarcasm that is born of legitimate fear.

Fern's Hungry Child is right. Talk is cheap. Only if her Adult can stay in *regular* touch with her and *show* her that her needs can be appropriately met is there a chance for her Nourished Child to emerge. Like you, Fern is taking baby steps here. She's just getting her balance, discovering whether she'll falter or make it across the room. It's far too early to tell whether she has developed the muscles and skills to trust herself to make it across.

Our goal this week has been to set the stage for you to stand on your own. One way to accomplish this goal is to assist you in accessing and using your Adult self in "reparenting" your Hungry Child. The Food for Thought exercises that follow are designed to help your Adult keep you from giving up on yourself. As an introduction to your daily exercises, I'd like to quote from Virginia Satir, a distinguished family therapist who died a few years ago:

"In a nurturing family, it is easy to pick up the message that human life and human feelings are more important than anything else. These parents see themselves as leaders, not bosses, and they see their job as primarily one of teaching their child how to be truly human in all situations."

> *We carry our homes within us, which enables us to fly.*
>
> —JOHN CAGE

FOOD FOR THOUGHT

WEEK TEN

Days One Through Seven

I want you to carry with you at all times the photograph you wrote to this week. When the old tapes start and you feel the urge to turn to

There's one blessing only, the source and cornerstone of beatitude—confidence in self.

—SENECA

food, instead, look at the picture and try to use the dual-handed technique to exchange brief notes with the Child in that picture. If you find yourself flooded with feelings, see if you can dialogue your way back and forth through them. Here are some scenarios I've included to get the ball rolling.

Day One

You've worked hard all day. You're exhausted. Nothing specific is bothering you, but as you look at the fish you've taken out to defrost, you begin to fantasize about ordering in a pizza.

Hungry Child: _____

_____

Adult: _____

_____

Hungry Child: _____

_____

Adult: _____

_____

Day Two

You've just picked up your car at the repair shop. The bill was more than you expected. As you pull into your driveway, you realize that the car is still not working properly.

Hungry Child: _____

_____

Adult: _____

_____

Hungry Child: _____

_____

Adult: _____

_____

Day Three

Your birthday is coming to an end and someone very close to you hasn't called.

Hungry Child: _____

_____

Adult: _____

_____

Hungry Child: _____

_____

Adult: _____

_____

Day Four

You've spent hours laboring over the stove or on some project at work. The person or people on the receiving end greet your efforts with comments like "Didn't we have chicken on Sunday?" or "Thanks, but I forgot to tell you we won't be needing that."

Hungry Child: _____

_____

Adult: _____

_____

Hungry Child: _____

_____

Adult: _____

_____

Be thine own palace, or the world's thy jail.

—JOHN DONNE

Day Five

You've been really focusing on what you put into your mouth. You're pleased with yourself for making smart choices. Eagerly, you step on the scale. Your weight is up a pound.

Hungry Child: _____
_____

Adult: _____
_____

Hungry Child: _____
_____

Adult: _____
_____

Day Six

You've spent a day working at your computer. Suddenly something happens—you don't know what—and all your work has disappeared. It's two hours later and you can't retrieve it.

Hungry Child: _____
_____

Adult: _____
_____

Hungry Child: _____
_____

Adult: _____
_____

Day Seven

You're at a party. You barely know anyone. The buffet table beckons.

Hungry Child: _____

_____

Adult: _____

_____

Hungry Child: _____

_____

Adult: _____

_____

Weekly Checklist

___ 1. Did you complete the visualization and writing exercises in this chapter?

___ 2. Did you complete the Food for Thought writing exercises?

Connections

❧

This week you will discover that you don't have to be religious to use rituals to save your soul.

❧

There is no meaning to life except the meaning man gives his life by the unfolding of his powers.

—ERICH FROMM

I'm hoping that you came out of last week, including the Food for Thought exercises, with your Adult, Loving Parent, and Nourished Child playing more dominant roles on your stage. This week I want to show you how these characters can work together to assist you in a new and most exciting way.

For many people who *are* religious, rituals play an essential role. Religions offer hundreds if not thousands of rituals to their followers, such as when a Catholic takes Communion, a Protestant couple baptizes their child, a Jewish woman lights Sabbath candles, a Muslim turns toward Mecca to pray, a Hindu prepares a funeral pyre, or a Buddhist chants. We know that rituals are a powerful force, but do we know why?

Mary: "To me, it's obvious. All the things I do in church reaffirm my belief. They keep me feeling connected with God. It's nice to feel that you're not alone, that there's something much bigger than you. Every element of the service, every ritual or rite, does that for me. They give me a sense of continuity."

Fern: "The only time I really go into a synagogue is for the High

Holy Days, Rosh Hashanah and Yom Kippur. I have a lot of mixed feelings about religion, but I guess what I like about the rituals is not so much that they bring me closer to a higher power, but that they are a reminder of my past. We always went as a family when I was growing up. Now, when I say the prayer for the dead, it's mainly for my father, and I can remember him sitting next to me and saying it for *his* father. There's something comforting about this for me. Maybe our compulsive eating is basically the same: It's a ritual that keeps us connected with our old script through our Hungry Child and Problematic Parent. Except in this instance, I think the rituals of the High Holy Days give me a very healthy connection."

Brendan: "Religious rituals are just the opposite for me. I vividly remember sitting next to my father in church on Sunday morning, him looking absolutely beatific, and me knowing how he terrorized our whole family the night before. Not to mention that he would punch me in the leg if I moved in my seat during the service. I mean, I understand that the church welcomes sinners, but in my father's case, it seemed so hypocritical. There was one ritual I *do* remember liking, though, if it really was a ritual. That was the putting up of the Christmas tree. For some reason, my father stayed relatively sober around Christmas, and each year he and I would go out and buy the tree together, carry it home, and decorate it. It was a real 'guy' thing. It's amazing how, in my anger at him, I had repressed this; he actually made many of the decorations himself. For all his problems, he was a very artistic person."

Brendan says he's not sure whether buying and putting up a Christmas tree qualifies as a ritual. In the strict religious sense, no. But in the broader sense of a "pattern of behavior performed in a prescribed manner," certainly. And in this larger arena, there literally is no end to the possibilities for ritualistic behavior. Fern, for example, cites the compulsive eating of the Hungry Child as a ritualistic form of behavior. How about you? In the space below, list up to five really *positive, nonreligious, non-food-related* activities you engage in, which in the broadest sense might qualify as rituals:

Keep in mind always the present you are constructing. It should be the future you want.

—ALICE WALKER

Rituals I Enjoy

1. _____
2. _____
3. _____
4. _____
5. _____

Here were some of the favorite rituals that Fern, Brendan, and Mary listed:

Fern: 1. Going to the Harvard–Yale football game every year.
            2. Watching "Sixty Minutes" every Sunday.
            3. Taking my stuffed dog to bed with me each night.
            4. Visiting my father's grave with my brother on the anniversary of his death.
            5. Paying my bills on the third Thursday of each month (I have no idea why!).

Brendan: 1. Clapping my hands at the end of any day when the market has gone up.
            2. Going to an AA meeting at least once a month.
            3. Dressing up like Santa at the office Christmas party.
            4. My annual reunion in Palm Springs with three high school buddies.
            5. The things I do every Saturday to keep my beloved BMW looking shipshape.

Mary: 1. Wearing something green on St. Patrick's Day.
            2. Volunteering at a homeless shelter once a month (since 1984).
            3. Spring cleaning.
            4. Making a baby quilt for each new grandchild (three so far).
            5. Being taken out to dinner on Mother's Day.

How did Fern's, Brendan's, and Mary's lists compare with your own? For all the differences, were there common denominators?

Mary: "Well, like the religious rituals, there seems to be something comforting about each of them."

Fern: "I agree. Whether it's watching Andy Rooney or holding Rosie, my stuffed dug, as I fall asleep each night, all these things are definitely comforting. There's that feeling of being connected that I talked about."

Brendan: "Same with me. I like things that keep me connected with people, even if it's not too close a connection. My *car* is actually like a person to me. It even has a name: Big Blue."

The feelings of comfort and connection that come from behaviors repeated over and over are beyond doubt the centerpiece of rituals. The human race seeks this out in events like the Olympics. Individual nations find it in their national holidays. In families, rituals can range from blowing out birthday candles to gathering at the same Vermont inn each fall for a reunion. As Fern, Brendan, and Mary make clear, rituals can provide great emotional satisfactions.

That's the good part. When your Hungry Child stuffs herself with food, when it engages in the ritual of compulsive eating, the result is quite different. But the underlying dynamics are much the same. As I said in the Introduction: When compulsive eaters talk about their *loss of connection* to themselves during a feeding frenzy, it is because they have been *reconnected* to a whole set of unconscious links between feelings and food.

It is this unconscious link between feelings and food that the ritual of our compulsive eating elicits. To help you, I want you to bring to the table one of the characters we've been talking about at length recently. That's right. Your Adult. If your Adult were to analyze the ritual of compulsive eating, what would she or he observe?

Fern: "If my Adult were onstage, as you put it, and not being critical, I guess it would make the point that the ritual *does* serve a purpose."

Brendan: "I don't mean to be a Problematic Parent, but how can you not be critical of something that's just an escape from feelings?"

Mary: "But it's not just an escape from feelings. My Adult tells me that the connection I make with being given cookies when I was a

Every exit has an entry somewhere else.

—PROVERB

kid—even if it was meant to sedate me—made me feel loved. That's more than an escape."

Brendan: "You're right. But I'm sure all of our Adults would also say that the only way the connection works now is keeping us in that old script."

Fern: "So how does our Adult get us out besides explaining all this?"

How indeed? How can our Adult get us out of a paradoxical trap in which our ritualistic compulsive eating simultaneously disconnects us from current feelings while reconnecting us unconsciously with past associations with feelings and food? How does our Adult rescue a Mary who looks to calm herself with food after being berated by her boss and in the process takes herself emotionally back to the nurturing quality food served for her as a child?

Mary: "I thought the idea was that my Adult helps me by giving me different thoughts about what happened with my supervisor, and that keeps my Hungry Child from taking over, which in turn keeps me out of that vicious cycle we talk about."

No single event can awaken within us a stranger totally unknown to us. To live is to be slowly born.

—ANTOINE DE SAINT-EXUPÉRY

Up to a point, our Adult can do exactly that. Mary, Fern, and Brendan are all reporting that as time goes by, the more they use their Adult this way, the better they feel about themselves and the better they're doing with compulsive eating. But like the end of any good drama, there's always some unfinished business to wrap up before the curtain descends. In the play about compulsive eating, that unfinished business is Brendan's comment way back in Week One: "I don't really need some negative event to set me off. I can binge regularly, and I can do it after I've had a perfectly fine day."

What are we to make of this? How does our Adult make sense of compulsive eating that seems to occur in the absence of stress? And even if it could make sense of it, how can it bail us out?

Fern: "I don't know about the second part of the puzzle, but I think I have the answer to the first part, at least for me. It's the realization I had that my big food issue is not just the way my mother controlled me with food, but the way my dad and I would have our secret raids on the refrigerator. That's a powerful, positive association I still seem to have."

"Powerful" may not be a strong enough word to convey the meaning of this connection for Fern. As she says, compulsive eating is not just a rebellion against her mother. It preserves the memory of her father, and not just in a general sense. In a family with a tradition of boys getting the parental spotlight, Fern's midnight sorties in the kitchen with her dad were the one arena in which brother Richie and Mom were out of the picture. In another family, a grown man might lovingly remember how he used to go hunting with his dad. In this family, a grown woman has wonderful associations with the way she and her dad used to go hunting for food.

And there's the rub. To ask Fern to take the meaning of this late-night ritual she and her dad shared and shove it into the garbage disposal would be the emotional equivalent of transporting a jungle animal to the seashore and asking it to survive. Like Fern, it would have no bearings. It would, in every sense, be lost.

Brendan: "But there's plenty of food along the shore. Maybe the animal would adapt."

Maybe. If she could find a way of rooting herself in this new environment, perhaps she could find new ways of "connecting" with food. Which is precisely what Fern, Mary, Brendan, and *you* will have to find a way to do if you want to permanently change your dysfunctional food relationship into one with healthy emotional roots.

The question is *how*. What kind of *action* can we take that will ensure our Adult self doesn't abandon us? This, I think, is our Adult's greatest challenge. In ancient Greek drama, at the end of the play, when the situation seemed beyond hope, a device called *deus ex machina* (literally, "God from machine") would be carried onto the stage. The device was a tall, wooden contraption at the top of which an actor playing a godlike figure would magically provide a solution. Unlike the characters in a Greek play, the rest of us have to rely on our own devices to create a desirable ending.

For Fern, it took a great deal of thought, but what her Adult finally came up with was creative and healing: "For a long time, thinking about the assignment left me feeling like I was trying to punch my way out of a paper bag. I knew by now that I had to deal with the connection I had with my father and food. I understood that it wasn't about food, but about love. I also was fully conscious by now that in

Discovery consists of seeing what everybody has seen and thinking what nobody has thought.

—ALBERT SZENT-GYÖRGYI VON NAGYRAPOLT

some way saying good-bye to my compulsive eating meant saying good-bye to my father. The problem was that I was in no way ready to say good-bye to the feelings that went with the way we bonded when I was a girl.

"Then it hit me. Maybe I didn't have to say good-bye to anything. If what my father and I did was in some way a ritual, maybe I could come up with another ritual that would work better for me. For a long time, I couldn't think of anything, but then my own *deus ex machina* miraculously appeared. And would you believe, it came packaged in an announcement from Nabisco!

"You see, when I was growing up, we had a kosher home, and that meant we couldn't eat all kinds of things. But the one my father would talk most about was Oreo cookies. They were his forbidden fruit. He had never had one, and sometimes he used to jokingly say, 'Oh boy, what I wouldn't do for an Oreo. Some people might walk a mile for a Camel. Me, I'd walk a mile for an Oreo.'

"And then a few weeks ago I pick up the paper and there's a story that Nabisco is starting to make kosher Oreos! Incredible! And my first thought? No surprise: 'If only Daddy had been alive.' I couldn't get that thought out of my head. And then later that day on the bus coming home from work, it hit me. Just like that.

"In my list of rituals I liked, I mentioned going with my brother to my father's grave on the anniversary of his death. Mom doesn't like to go. She says it's too painful. But Richie and I go and we stay awhile, and just before we leave, we put a pebble on the headstone. It's a symbolic way of saying we were there.

"Last Saturday, I went by myself. There was no special occasion, and I didn't tell anyone I was going. Before I went, I bought a bag of kosher Oreos. I had really thought about this, and when I arrived at his plot, I opened up the bag and counted out seventeen cookies. That's the number of pounds I've lost so far. I took the cookies and put them on top of the headstone, like the pebbles. I told my father that they were from me. I told him to enjoy them. And I left. On the way out, I stopped and gave the rest of the bag to a cemetery worker.

"I can't tell you how good this made me feel. And I assure you, I'm not delusional. I know that birds and squirrels, not my father, will actually eat the cookies. It doesn't matter. I feel like I've kept my relationship with my father alive in a great way. I know doing something once doesn't make it a ritual, but I plan to continue to do this, maybe

We are not permitted to choose the frame of our destiny. But what we put into it is ours.

—DAG HAMMARSKJÖLD

every few months in the beginning. And except for this group, I'm not going to tell anyone else. This is a little secret between my father and me."

What do you think of Fern's ritual? I was certainly impressed by its originality, but even more by the way Fern managed to create something that directly maintained the emotional connection with her father *through* food, but turned it around so that the loving tie was preserved through a *noneating* event. Uneaten cookies. A neat emotional sleight of hand!

When Brendan came up with a ritual to help himself, he never had to leave home. Where his Adult took him emotionally, however, turned out to be just as far afield and just as surprising:

"When I began to think about me and food, of course, all that came to mind was my mother using food to comfort me or sedate me or whatever she did with food, given the fact that my father was an alcoholic bully and she wasn't going to kick him out. So what am I supposed to do? Find some other ritual to help me connect with my mother besides comforting myself with food. Hey, I already have lots of ways to do that. So what's the point?

"My Adult really came through for me while I was at an AA meeting. Usually I sit there and listen to others talk and maybe talk myself, and regardless of what's said, there's a value to just being there. Like coming to these workshops, it helps me stay focused. On this particular night, I suddenly had this other thought. It went something like this: Why are you here? Answer: Because you're an alcoholic. Question: And whom did you inherit your alcoholism from? Answer: Your father. Question: So that was your connection with your father? Answer: You mean that we had the same disease? Fine. But I was not the same kind of alcoholic he was. Alcohol was bad for me, but when I drank I was happy and loving. My father was an angry, mean, abusive drunk. Question: Right, but like it or not, drinking was a connection the two of you had? Answer: So now I don't drink and I've lost my connection? Because if that's what you're getting at, let me tell you, I don't need any connection with my father. End of story.

"Or so I thought. And then, I'm not sure exactly when, I realized that this was a lie. For all these years, I've been telling myself that when he was alive or now that he's dead, all I wanted from my father was to

The final forming of a person's character lies in their own hands.

—ANNE FRANK

The winds and the waves
are always on the side of
the ablest navigators.

—EDWARD GIBBON

be his polar opposite. And as hard as it was for me to admit to myself, I realized that *every* boy must want a connection with his father, no matter who or what his father is or was. Saying it now, it seems so obvious. When I first had this thought, though, I felt weak and ashamed.

"Happily, my Adult intervened just in time and it rescued me. It did this by assuring me that it took strength to admit that I might want some connection, that this is what decorating the Christmas tree with my father was all about. In my anger, it was a memory I had consciously forgotten about, but the memory was there all along; tucked away, but clearly there. So maybe this was the time to let it out. Maybe I could allow that and still feel safe.

"I had no idea where all this would lead me, but it's amazing how the human mind operates. What happened was that one night last week, I stopped at the gym after work and then came home. Usually I'd watch a little TV at this hour and then go to bed. This particular night I had energy, probably because I had exercised, and I felt like I needed to do something. So what did I do? Not even consciously, I found myself taking some paper and a pen out of my desk drawer. At first, I was just doodling. The next thing I knew, I was drawing pictures of funny, happy little creatures, and it just became clear that I was going to turn them into three-dimensional objects and use them next year to decorate my Christmas tree. My father had artistic aptitude. Alcoholism is not the only thing I inherited from him. So that's what I plan to turn into my ritual. An AA meeting a month. A Christmas ornament a month. I like that. I'm not sure I want to think too much about *why* I like my rituals so much, but I'll give it a shot. I guess food is actually at the heart of my ritual because my mother used to sedate me with it after my father was abusive, verbally or physically. He scared the hell out of all of us, and my compulsive eating probably takes me back to that time. So maybe, by connecting with him in a different way, I feel less intimidated. It's true. Whenever I think about my ritual, I actually feel stronger. I also seem to feel less compelled to reach for food."

What are your thoughts about Brendan's ritual? At first glance, the one he settled on, making Christmas decorations, seems unrelated to food. At second glance, it seems to me very much related. In creating his ritual, Brendan made two extremely important breakthroughs. Consciously, he realized that despite everything, he *did* want a connection with his father. Perhaps unconsciously, he understood that Mom's "sedative" food followed Dad's anger and violence. Brendan's father *was* scary. Changing the food-fear connection with him to one that puts Brendan in a better, more *empowered* relationship through Christmas decorations is another nail in the coffin of his compulsive eating. No wonder Brendan says, "I like that."

Finally we come to Mary. If she puts herself last in her own family, it's certainly not my intention to do so here. It's just that I think that what Mary has been struggling with most of her life may have a special relevance to *you*. And the ritual she settled on, which had neither the dramatic flair of Fern's nor the unexpected twist of Brendan's, was, I think, profoundly perfect for Mary:

"I really struggled with this. I'm not a particularly creative person, but I don't think that was the only reason. It was more that every time I thought about what a ritual might be, I ended up back at square one, by which I mean that the ideas didn't seem like they would work.

"The first area I concentrated on was my grandmother and the food she would give me that made me feel loved. I just couldn't think of anything to do around that. Then I thought I was really getting somewhere when I began to think about my mother. I've mentioned that she wasn't really available and that she had these nervous breakdowns from time to time. I've often felt guilty that I couldn't somehow have helped her, even though I rationally know I was a kid. In light of things I've read as an adult, I've also wondered whether her depressions weren't related in some way to my father not being around much and how, like me, she had great difficulty expressing her feelings and her needs. I don't really know if it was about that or if it was biological, but like I said, I've often felt guilty because I was much closer to my grandmother than to my mother.

"So the thought occurred to me: Maybe it would be healing if I worked some way with the mentally ill. I could get a little more training and become a psychiatric nurse. I could do volunteer work. Or—and I thought this was really clever—I could make a connection between my grandmother and my mother and bake cookies for someplace that works with emotionally disturbed people.

"Just when I was congratulating myself, this voice popped into my head. It may sound like the Problematic Parent, but in truth it was my Adult. And the voice said, 'Mary, there you go again. You're about to

Freedom is a condition of mind, and the best way to secure it is to breed it.

—ELBERT HUBBARD

start providing for people again. That's what you always do. This is not the way.' And the voice was right. And I was back at square one.

"I think because it was my Adult speaking, I didn't give up. I just kept thinking, and what came to mind first was the item on my good-ritual list about being taken out for Mother's Day. I really do look forward to that. What flashed into my head next was how I asked my husband to get me a piece of pie on Thanksgiving, and how unusual that was for me.

"As I thought about these things, I realized how much I enjoy it when someone does something nice for me. And this is where so much of what we've been talking about suddenly came together: 'Mary,' I said to myself, 'if you like being taken care of, why can't you do that for yourself? Giving to yourself would really be something new, and if you need to justify it, just tell yourself it's a gift your mother couldn't give herself and you're doing it for the both of you.'

"So here's my ritual: I have started something called Mary's Treat of the Month Club. Each month, I plan to give myself a different treat. All by myself. Just for me. Last week was the first. I went and had a massage. It was the first I ever had. I felt so guilty beforehand that I almost canceled the appointment, but I forced myself to go and I loved it! I'm already thinking about next month."

The first thing Mary deserves is great credit for not falling into the same old script by creating a ritual that would have kept her role intact as the provider for others. Once Mary's Adult realized that all her early ideas were taking her in that direction, Mary hit on an idea that I think showed great courage. Giving oneself treats may not seem like a big deal to some, but for Mary it had always been equated with selfishness. To begin to do so now—to give herself *healthy* treats publicly instead of *mistreating* herself privately with compulsive eating—is a huge step in the *right* direction.

Fern, Brendan, and Mary all said that their rituals were not a total answer, but an important tool in their battle against compulsive eating. None was able to explain completely why, but I believe the answer lies largely in what each said at the beginning of this week about rituals in general. Mary talked about the *continuity* rituals provided. Fern focused on the *healthy connection* she experienced. Brendan described unearthing a *repressed* memory. The rituals they then created combined all of these elements. In the process, Brendan, Fern, and Mary were en-

That is what learning is. You suddenly understand something you've understood all your life, but in a new way.

—DORIS LESSING

couraged to *consciously substitute* a healthy ritual, which allowed them to *feel* something important, for the *unconscious* ritual of compulsive eating, which served to bury feelings that no longer needed to be hidden.

FOOD FOR THOUGHT

WEEK ELEVEN

Day One

Go back and analyze the ritual Fern came up with for herself. Write down any elements of it, specific or general, that might work for you.

_____

_____

_____

_____

The mind is a strange machine which can combine the material offered to it in the most astonishing ways.

—BERTRAND RUSSELL

Day Two

Go back and analyze Brendan's ritual. Write down any elements, specific or general, that might work for you.

_____

_____

_____

_____

Day Three

Go back and analyze Mary's ritual. Write down any elements, specific or general, that might work for you.

_____

_____

_____

_____

Day Four

Focusing on your own life, and using anything you've learned from

Fern, Brendan, and Mary, think of a ritual that might therapeutically address your emotional relationship with food.

_____

_____

_____

_____

Day Five

Write down why you think the ritual you created in Day Four might really work for you. If you're having second thoughts, write them down here and see if you can come up with a ritual that might serve you better.

_____

_____

_____

_____

We have to do with the past only as we can make it useful to the present and the future.

—FREDERICK DOUGLASS

Day Six

Perform your ritual.

Day Seven

Write down all your thoughts and feelings about what you did in Day Six. If you were unable to perform your ritual, describe why. If you did, but discovered that it didn't work, go back to Day Five and keep thinking. Your goal is not to pass a creativity test. It is to give yourself a gift.

_____

_____

_____

_____

Weekly Checklist

____ 1. Are you using your Adult voice to walk you through your difficult moments?

____ 2. Did you complete your Food for Thought writing exercises?

WEEK TWELVE

Beginning Again

❧

We shall not cease from exploration.
And the end of all our exploring
Will be to arrive where we started
And know the place for the first time.
          —T. S. Eliot

Our first goal for this, our last week together, is to go back to where *we* started on our journey. I want to try to recapture some moments we shared that first week we met. I'd like us to revisit some of our major stopping points along the way.

❧

As for the future, your task is not to foresee, but to enable it.

—Antoine de Saint-Exupéry

Brendan: "Well, one thing that's obvious to me is how much Fern and Mary have changed over the past twelve weeks. I don't mean the obvious physical changes as a result of their weight loss. I'm talking more about personality things. Fern, I don't want you to take this the wrong way, but when I first met you, you scared the hell out of me. I thought that one wrong word out of me and you'd be down my throat. And now, you're no shrinking violet or anything, but you seem so much softer . . . warmer . . . less angry.

"And Mary, when you first came in, you were almost invisible. When you spoke, it was practically a whisper. I had to strain to hear you. And look at you today! I don't mean to make you self-conscious, but you're wearing red. You're definitely visible. And your voice has become much more vibrant. I think it's great. There's such a big difference in both you and Fern.

"As for me, well, I have not been as *judicious* as Fern in working the program, and I certainly have not been as *religious* as Mary in doing the weekly assignments, but I will say that I have lost over twenty pounds, and I realize that despite my initial skepticism and resistance, I can see some pretty dramatic changes in myself as well."

Fern: "It's interesting that Brendan finds me warmer and softer. I've been hearing words to that effect from other people as well. At first, I have to admit that I was very ambivalent about this kind of feedback. I know it was meant as a compliment, but it made me feel too vulnerable, like people were looking at me too closely. But as I started to be a little kinder to myself, other people's comments have become a lot easier to take. So thank you for noticing, Brendan! I realize over these past several weeks that not only have I gained insight into my own *self*, but I have developed a much keener understanding of others as well.

"One of the biggest changes I've noticed about you in the last twelve weeks, Brendan, is that you don't joke around as much. You're still a funny guy, but I no longer see you using humor as one of your *defensive dwarfs* to protect you when you are feeling uncomfortable with the material being discussed in the group. So I think that, like me, you're much more approachable, but in a different way. You seem much more real to me, and I really like that.

"As for you, Mary, what can I say? What a transformation! You talk to everyone. You have a new haircut. You wear colorful, fitted clothes. It's like your fearful, hiding, Hungry Child has come out of the closet with a whole new wardrobe. Truly amazing."

Mary: "I'm grateful for what you've said, Brendan and Fern. And if I were to take this 'new' me to the extreme, I'd say keep those compliments coming. You know, when I look back and remember that first day I walked in here, I vividly recall how self-conscious and inadequate I felt. I literally wanted to hide under this table. When I see myself now, it's almost scary. I know I have come a long way over the past three months, but I also know that all of this is still very new to me. It's going to take lots more practice before I can say, 'Look, Ma, no hands.'

"I want to say that I notice just as many changes in the two of you.

The future belongs to those who believe in the beauty of their dreams.

—ELEANOR ROOSEVELT

Fern, I completely agree with Brendan when he says you seem much less angry, much more approachable. I was intimidated by both you and Brendan in the beginning. In different ways, you were each so forceful. Now I feel very close to both of you. I think we are all less defensive and more real. I pray each night that we all continue to stay on track."

The *outer* changes Brendan, Fern, and Mary have been talking about all are reflections of the significant *internal* changes they have started to make. A dramatic shift has begun to occur in how dominant a role each of their characters plays in their respective scripts. The healthier characters—the Adult, Loving Parent, and Nourished Child—are more center stage, more in sync with one another. We see this evidenced by the greater warmth and softness in Fern, the more outgoing nature in Mary, and the less comically camouflaged side of Brendan. And as their Hungry Child has begun to recede from the spotlight, so has their compulsive eating. When I asked the three of them to write down some thoughts about the specifics of their emotional voyage, here's how they responded:

Mary: "I think the most important thing I've discovered over the weeks is that it's my Hungry Child that's front and center in my head when I'm in my *vicious cycle* and eating compulsively. I also gained an increasing awareness about the ways in which expectations, rewards, food, and emotional needs have unconsciously fueled my self-destructive script. It's hard for me to put all these elements together as neatly as the pieces of some quilt I'm making, but I know for sure that my compulsive eating has created a wedge which kept me disconnected from others and from myself. I think I know much more about how that developed out of my childhood. In the language we've used in this program, my Adult has helped teach me that it's safe for me to be visible at this time in my life. It's okay to have needs.

"For me, the insights I've had these weeks have been important, but what's even more helpful are the concrete skills I've developed to counteract my old script, to keep me out of the *vicious cycle*. The more I have a healthy internal family, the more inner harmony I feel, the less compulsive eating I do. You were right, Marilyn. In the first few weeks of the program, the intensity and duration and frequency of my binges began to subside. It seems almost eerie, but in the last few weeks, I haven't binged at all."

Every cloud has a silver lining.

—UNKNOWN

❧

Fern: "What I remember about my first few weeks here is that even though I was really desperate to do something about my weight, I still was very skeptical or cynical about this program. It wasn't personal. It was the way I was about everything. All the other weight-loss methods I had tried hadn't worked. Endless years of therapy hadn't helped. So in the beginning when I saw Mary pull out her notebook and write down every word you said, and complete all her homework assignments so meticulously, I'm ashamed to admit that I actually felt superior to her, like she was trying to be the teacher's pet or something. When I tell you now that Mary has turned out to be an inspiration to me, I think I'm saying as much about my own changes as about hers. Something very different has happened to me here, something very special. Finally, for the first time, it all began to make sense to me. Like everyone else, I discovered that food and eating served many functions for me. On some level, I think I already knew that food was a way I kept the power struggle going between my mother and me. The discovery that food also kept alive my connection with my dad was probably the biggest realization of my life.

"As valuable to me as these insights were in helping me understand *why* I compulsively overate, the truth is that they would not have been enough. One of the things I learned the hard way in therapy is that understanding doesn't necessarily produce change. What this program has given me beyond enlightenment are tools. Once I began to get over my resistance and started doing the exercises and working sincerely with the different players in my head, things really did start to change. And the beauty of it all is that I've been losing weight without all the pain in the you-know-what of weighing every ounce of food, or taking dangerous diet pills, or exercising myself to death. I'm not feeling deprived. In fact, quite the opposite. I'm feeling good, inside and out. For me, 'diet' has become a four-letter word. It's still early in the game, but if I can hold on to what I've learned here, I'll be truly taking care of myself for the first time."

Brendan: "I've often felt a little guilty sitting here each week and kind of listening but not really listening. Sometimes I would doodle or do the crossword puzzle while I waited for my turn to speak. There were times when I was more absorbed in thinking of something

❧

Our greatest weakness lies in giving up. The most certain way to succeed is always to try one more time.

—THOMAS EDISON

funny to say than in paying attention to whoever else was speaking. Some weeks I didn't do the Food for Thought exercises, or didn't do all of them. In the past, I would have said all these things by way of telling you and myself what a failure I am. But that's not what I feel now. Maybe that's because that would be my Hungry Child and Problematic Parent doing the talking, and you wouldn't want that now, would you?

"Seriously, I'm not going to beat up on myself because here it is, Week Twelve, and I'm still in the program, and I've lost quite a few pounds, actually, and I've been going to the gym, and all in all I'm feeling kind of bullish about myself (and not just because I'm a stockbroker!). I'm not going to review all the insights I've had about myself and food here, other than saying how aware I've become of the relationship in my *psyche* between food, alcohol, fear, and emotional sedation. The exercises we did in the group gave me the opportunity to get in touch with some of my deeply hidden feelings and recollections of my past. That, in itself, gave me a real sense of liberation. Other than that, I want to say that I'm thinking more and more these days about what you called the defensive dwarfs. I don't think any of them had the name Jokey, but that's definitely been the name of my biggest one. I think I'm beginning to really understand that I can be funny at times without using humor to hide from myself or others. That's a big, big change for me."

Persistence and determination are omnipotent.

—CALVIN COOLIDGE

How about you? Take a few minutes here to reflect on the discoveries and changes you've made over the past twelve weeks. Jot them down in the space below:

_____

_____

_____

_____

Mary, Fern, and Brendan all have experienced some truly remarkable awakenings during their twelve weeks together. They have addressed the dark roots of their compulsive eating, first by understanding that the seeds were planted in their early childhood and grew out of an unconscious, insatiable quest to fulfill an *unmet* or *inappropriately met* early developmental need. An unmet need that repeatedly reveals itself through each individual life script. A script that plays itself out in observable behaviors and consequences expressed in patterns of a "repetition compulsion," the vicious cycle.

As you may already know, this workbook was designed to allow you to probe below your intellectual and other psychological defenses to tap these unmet "child" needs that fuel your compulsive-eating patterns. During this process, you not only became aware of the inner workings of your life drama, but your growing consciousness helps you to effectively use the tools you've been acquiring to redirect your internal world to a level of wholeness and completeness. These corrective emotional experiences result in a gradual elimination of your compulsive-eating symptoms, leading to the body-weight normalization witnessed and expressed by Mary, Fern, and Brendan.

The goal now, at this stage of your recovery, is for you to make a renewed commitment to maintaining and sustaining the dramatic changes you've made so far. Before we say good-bye, then, *my* goal is to leave you with some final food for thought. I feel now the way I always do at the end of a workshop—like a mother sending her children off to camp. The duffel bags have been loaded onto the bus. There is a mix of joyous anticipation and anxiety in the air. And even though there have been months of careful preparation for this moment, Mom just can't help herself. As the bus starts to move slowly away, she is running alongside it, waving, throwing kisses, shouting reassuring words, and getting in one last "And don't forget to . . ."

If this week marks the end of one relationship, I hope it simultaneously heralds the beginning of a new one, both with yourself and with the world around you. Like any new relationship, yours is still in the fragile stages of development and will need continued support for the foundation you have been building. The tools I want to offer you now are guaranteed to give you that support. Use them and you will keep your house safe from the destructive storms of compulsive eating.

When I asked Fern, Brendan, and Mary what tools they thought would be most helpful to them, here's what *they* said:

Fern: "Without a doubt, always being conscious of that 'internal' family we have been working with. I have to admit that when I first heard you talking about the Hungry Child and the Problematic Parent, I was skeptical. But it's true. Those two, along with the Loving Parent, Adult, and Nourished Child *are* the separate characters that play in my

To be alive at all involves some risk.

—HAROLD MACMILLAN

head . . . I guess in all of our heads. And every time I stay in touch with my Loving Parent and Adult, I come out fine."

Brendan: "Same for me. I would only add that as hard as it has been at times for me to regularly do my Food for Thought exercises, they're really helpful when I do. So I plan to go back and keep doing them the way I now keep going back to the gym. It might help if I thought of the exercises as my emotional workout."

Mary: "I agree with what Fern and Brendan said. For me, I think another thing that will really help at this point is finding some kind of support group. Maybe with a couple of friends or starting a group or something. I have such a tendency to keep things bottled up inside me that I think it will be important if I can continue to share what I've been learning here with others."

Take a few moments to formulate the most important things you might do to stay on course in the weeks and months to come. Take your time, then jot them down in the space below:

_____
_____
_____
_____

By now you know implicitly that what you have just heard Fern, Brendan, and Mary say is their Adult talking. Their Adult with some Loving Parent thrown in for good measure. When your Adult is center stage, it will continue to provide you with food for life. It will do this by addressing your basic three "food" categories: your *physical needs;* your *spiritual needs* and your *social needs.* Let's take them one at a time.

FOOD FOR LIFE

My Physical Needs

Keep your Adult active and it will keep you asking and answering questions like these:

1. How much sleep do I need each night to keep myself well rested and healthy?_____

The desire accomplished is sweet to the soul.

—PROVERBS 13:19

If I'm not getting enough, how will I restructure my day and evening to get this need met?

_____

_____

_____

_____

2. Am I getting enough exercise each day to keep my heart and musculoskeletal system strong and fit so I can carry on my activities of daily living with ease and enjoyment?_____
Do I need a medical checkup first to see if I have any special problems?_____
Would it help me to have a few sessions with a personal trainer first to help me get started?_____

Realistically, how can I incorporate an activity plan for myself into my daily schedule? Whether it's taking a walk during my lunch break, signing up for an exercise class, or doing sit-ups at home, what combination of activities can I commit to that are varied, pleasurable, and, most important, within my means to accomplish? Take some time to sketch out a practical weekly plan. Don't forget to incorporate downtime.

Sunday:_____

_____

Monday:_____

_____

Tuesday: _____

_____

Wednesday:_____

_____

Thursday: _____

_____

Friday: _____

_____

Saturday:_____

_____

3. Are my body's nutritional needs being met?_____ Am I getting enough fruits, grains, high-protein foods, and vegetables?_____

If you surrendered to the air, you could ride it.

—TONI MORRISON

Am I making wholesome foods available for me to choose from?_____ Should I be cutting down or eliminating caffeine and alcohol?_____ If I don't know the answer to these questions, should I be reading up on the subject or sitting down with a professional nutritionist to educate myself and put together an eating program that works for my *particular* body?_____ Am I using my internal biological cues to tell me when my body needs to be fueled?_____ If I'm having trouble, will I go back to the Hunger Awareness Worksheet to help me refocus?_____ Am I drinking six to eight glasses of *water* each day, the recommended amount for my fluid needs to be met?_____ Will I carry bottled water around with me?_____ What's my game plan to make sure I let water do its many wonders? To protect me from confusing thirst with hunger? _____

My Spiritual Needs

Staying connected with your inner self requires the same kind of regular maintenance as keeping your car well tuned. If you value yourself, you will certainly put together a good internal maintenance plan. One way of checking under the hood is to regularly ask yourself questions like these:

Do I spend some time with myself each day to make sure I remain connected with my Adult?_____ Is my Adult and Loving Parent "feeding" my Hungry Child what she or he needs on a regular basis to feel like a Nourished Child?_____ What steps can I take to be sure my Child voice is heard?_____ Is there a special place I can go on a regular basis to center myself and rejuvenate my soul? A Park? A Lake? A church? Choose one place where you can regularly check in with yourself. It can be your own backyard. A special tree, your garden, a favorite room. But designate a place as your own and go there to commune with yourself and nourish your Hungry Child._____

How can I structure my day to make sure that I have enough time to do these things? When are the best times for me on weekdays? On weekends?_____

Within you there is a stillness and a sanctuary to which you can retreat at any time and be yourself.

—HERMANN HESSE

Develop a weekly plan for yourself below. List the things you will do on a daily basis to give voice to your feelings and maintain an inner connection.

Sunday:_____
_____

Monday:_____
_____

Tuesday: _____
_____

Wednesday:_____
_____

Thursday: _____
_____

Friday: _____
_____

Saturday:_____
_____

❧

Success is a journey, not a destination.

—BEN SWEETLAND

Many of the exercises you have done in *The Hunger Within* can continue to be valuable tools for you in the months and years to come. Below is a list of some of the most important ones. You will want to come back to this list frequently and work with whatever tool or tools you need at any given time.

Tools:
1. Revisit my *genogram* from time to time to stay in touch with the roots of my core image and compulsive eating.
2. Keep checking in on my internal family or cast. Think in terms of the five characters: *Hungry Child, Nourished Child, Problematic Parent, Loving Parent, Adult.* Be able to identify at all times which ones are occupying center stage.
3. Frame my *child photograph* and display it in a special place. Talk or write to that child whenever she or he needs to hear from me. Use my nondominant hand to get replies.
4. Listen to my *feelings.* They are an expression of my needs and provide me with the information I need to keep myself nurtured and fulfilled.
5. Use self-talk to keep lines of *internal communication* open. Do that

by going back to the Vicious Cycle chart. Follow the loop from *event* to *thoughts* to *feelings* to *behaviors* to *consequences*. When I'm having negative feelings, use my Adult to rescue the thoughts my Hungry Child is having.

6. I will go back from time to time and do the *string exercise* in Week Five to remind myself of how my thinking can be negatively distorted.

7. Keep a periodic tally of the *strokes* and *put-downs* I receive and give myself to make sure I am not operating out of my tired old script.

8. If I find myself going into a trancelike state and bingeing, eat in front of a *mirror* again to help me reconnect with myself.

9. Try to assess why my internal Snow White really needs to cling to one of the Seven Dwarfs (defense mechanisms) at any given time.

10. Remember that the scariest word in the English language is *change*. Appreciate that fact at times when I think I'm making U-turns to my past or going too slowly in the right direction.

*I came,
I saw, I conquered.*

—JULIUS CAESAR

My Social Needs

As you get your act together and take it on the road, developing and maintaining healthy connections with those around you is vitally important. Here are a few things you can do to help you stay connected to those around you:

1. Do I have a supportive outside network of people who encourage and respect my needs?
List the current roster of meaningful people in your life. It may include a person from your clergy, friends, family, etc.

My supportive outside network: _____
_____

2. Are there too few names on my list?_____ Too many?_____ Do enough relationships provide me with the support I need? _____ Are enough of my relationships mutually positive and supportive?_____ Are too many of them draining or one-way streets?_____

3. Here are some strategies I can use to create and enhance good relationships in my life:

_____

_____

_____

_____

4. Here are some strategies I can use to minimize or protect myself from those relationships that are negative or hurtful:

_____

_____

_____

_____

5. If my external support system is too limited, do I need to join some kind of support group?_____ Would it help me to get individual counseling?_____ Is there a religious group I might join or become more active in?_____ Other group or organization?_____ Which ones might I try out? _____

_____

When other people push your buttons and you find yourself drowning in your old script, here are some specific tools to help you stay afloat:

• I can take a "time-out," walk away from the person or situation, and regroup.

• I can analyze what it is about the person or situation that has triggered my response. Going back and rereading *The Hunger Within,* especially my own notes, can help my analysis.

• I will take as my motto the advice offered by Ophelia's father in *Hamlet:* "To thine own self be true." I will find my own voice in relationships. I will listen to it.

Of all the relationships you choose to have, I hope that the ones you've established with Fern, Brendan, and Mary will be among them. It would be *my* wish that you think of them from time to time as you continue your own journey. It would be *their* wish that I run now alongside your bus as it leaves for camp and that I shout these last words from them:

Fern: "Be patient with yourself. You're going to have
          relapses. Nobody's perfect. This is a process that takes
          a long time. Don't beat up on yourself. Don't give up
          on yourself."

Brendan: "Turn yourself into a blue-chip stock that keeps
          increasing in value. Don't be afraid. Don't let a day
          go by without laughing or making someone laugh."

Mary: "I'd like to leave you with an old Irish blessing: 'May
          the road rise up to meet you. May the wind be
          always at your back. May the sun shine warm upon
          your face. May the rain fall soft upon your fields. And
          until we meet again, may God hold you in the palm
          of His hand.' "

*But now all I need in
order to have a future, is
to design a future I can
manage to get inside of.*

—FRANCINE JULIAN CLARK

There is only one you.
And you will walk this path only once.
Make it the best journey it can be.

Good Luck and Best Wishes!

Suggested Reading

❧

Here is a list of readings to assist you on your road to recovery.

Beattie, Melody. *Beyond Codependency.* San Francisco: Harper and Row, 1989. A recovery book for mastering the art of self-care.

———. *The Language of Letting Go.* San Francisco: Harper and Row, 1990. A book of daily meditations.

Bradshaw, John. *Healing the Shame That Binds You.* Deerfield Beach, Fla.: Health Communications, Inc., 1988. Understanding the feelings of the Hungry Child.

———. *The Family.* Deerfield Beach, Fla.: Health Communications, Inc., 1988. An in-depth look at the role one's family plays in precipitating inner disconnection.

Breathnach, Sarah Ban. *Simple Abundance.* New York: Warner Books, Inc., 1995. A daybook of inspirational affirmations.

Burns, M.D., David D. *Feeling Good—The New Mood Therapy.* New York: Avon Books, 1980. A close analysis of destructive messages that push us into our vicious cycle.

Chopich, Erika J., and Paul, Margaret. *Healing Your Aloneness.* San Francisco: Harper and Row, 1990. A profound look at the cause of one's inner pain.

Jeffers, Susan. *Feel the Fear and Do It Anyway.* New York: Harcourt Brace

Jovanovich, 1987. Understanding what it means to face our fears and move beyond them.

Miller, Alice. *The Drama of the Gifted Child.* New York: HarperCollins Publishers, Inc., 1994. Reclaiming one's life through discovering one's own needs.

Roth, Geneen. *When Food Is Love.* New York: Dutton Publishing Company, Inc., 1991. A compelling personal account of the author's own struggle in her relationship with food.

Acknowledgments

❧

I would like to extend my heartfelt gratitude to those involved in making this book a reality:

Dr. Brett Seabury at the University of Michigan, who, through his creative teaching style, inspired me to develop my experientially based workshops and subsequent workbook. Xavier Pi-Sunyer, M.D., Medical Director, and all the staff at St. Luke's–Roosevelt Hospital for their ongoing encouragement and support. My agent, Nick Ellison, and Christina Harcar for their support in getting this project off the ground. Philip Ross, for his help in writing and transforming my twelve-week workshop into a workbook format. My editor, Betsy Lerner, and to her assistant Matthew Ellis, for her invaluable editorial guidance. Richard Elam, for the graphics layout and design work of all worksheets and charts. Ellie Filanowski and Eileen Sierra for providing their professional word-processing services. Greg Gulia, for his legal assistance and guidance.

A special thanks to my family: my parents, Greg and Rose Migliore; my sisters, Carol and Nancy; my brother-in-law, Mike; my nephew, Nick. And to my close friend and colleague, Robin Ferris. Last but not least, I would like to extend my deepest appreciation to all of my workshop participants who, by courageously sharing their own stories, have given a voice to *Brendan, Mary,* and *Fern.*

About the Author

❧

Marilyn Ann Migliore is a certified nutritionist and psychotherapist who has worked as a group and individual counselor for people with eating disorders for more than twenty years. At the University of Michigan, where she completed her graduate degree and training, she was part of a multidisciplinary team that specialized in eating disorders. This experience laid the foundation for the development and implementation of her specialized workshops for compulsive eaters. Her work has been reported on national television and in various popular magazines. This book is founded on her successful workshops and is designed especially for the last-ditch dieter.